CSA
PRACTICE
CASES FOR THE
MRCGP

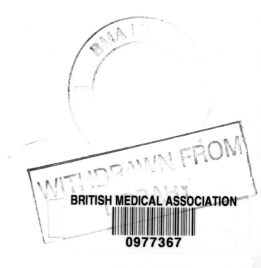

OTHER TITLES FROM SCION

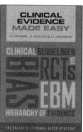

9781907904202

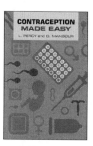

9781907904301

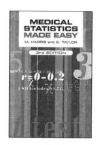

9781907904035

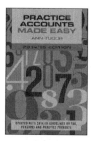

9781907904172

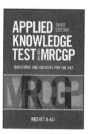

9781907904189

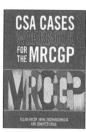

9781907904127

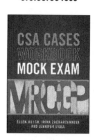

9781907904653

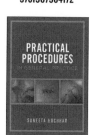

9781904842996

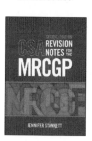

9781907904073

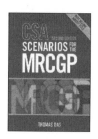

9781907904639

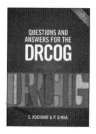

9781907904196

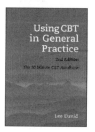

9781904842934

For more details see www.scionpublishing.com

CSA PRACTICE CASES FOR THE MRCGP

Prashini Naidoo

MBChB, MRCGP, DRCOG, DFFP, Dip Occ, MSc
GP in Oxfordshire

and

Sonali Bapat

MBBS, MRCGP
GP in Sussex

Scion

© **Scion Publishing Limited, 2016**

First published 2016

All rights reserved. No part of this book may be reproduced or transmitted, in any form or by any means, without permission.

A CIP catalogue record for this book is available from the British Library.

ISBN 978 1 907904 34 9

Scion Publishing Limited

The Old Hayloft, Vantage Business Park, Bloxham Road, Banbury OX16 9UX, UK

www.scionpublishing.com

Important Note from the Publisher

The information contained within this book was obtained by Scion Publishing Ltd from sources believed by us to be reliable. However, while every effort has been made to ensure its accuracy, no responsibility for loss or injury whatsoever occasioned to any person acting or refraining from action as a result of information contained herein can be accepted by the authors or publishers.

Readers are reminded that medicine is a constantly evolving science and while the authors and publishers have ensured that all dosages, applications and practices are based on current indications, there may be specific practices which differ between communities. You should always follow the guidelines laid down by the manufacturers of specific products and the relevant authorities in the country in which you are practising.

Although every effort has been made to ensure that all owners of copyright material have been acknowledged in this publication, we would be pleased to acknowledge in subsequent reprints or editions any omissions brought to our attention.

Registered names, trademarks, etc. used in this book, even when not marked as such, are not to be considered unprotected by law.

Typeset by Medlar Publishing Solutions Pvt Ltd, India

Printed in the UK

Contents

PART II

Preface

When candidates are asked what they want from practice cases in a CSA preparation book, some say they want cases with lots of background explanation and others want more succinct cases because they are easier to work through in the final few weeks before the exam. It is therefore difficult to get the balance right for everybody. However, we have tried to cater for everyone by writing a book of two halves:

- the first half of the book contains two CSA circuits of 13 cases per circuit – these cases contain lots of detail and are an ideal way to start preparing for the exam
- the second half of the book also contains two complete CSA circuits, but the cases are more concise and so ideal to work through as the real exam gets closer.

Part I

These 26 cases contain an extensive brief to the role-player. The advantage of this is that the role-player does not have to be a medical person; you could practise with someone at work or a spouse. The role-player, after a single reading of the script, can get into the skin of being that patient and consistently provide the cues and information needed for the doctor to appropriately manage the case. The doctor, looking at the role-player notes, also gets an idea of what it feels like to be the person with a medical issue. This helps to develop empathy.

The cases also contain an extensive list of questions and suggestions for the doctor. While some candidates may look at this list and become overwhelmed by the amount of detail given, others may see it as a model of what a good, experienced doctor should do. When it is broken down in this way, with all the detail, the candidate learns the various tasks and skills involved in being a competent and good GP.

Let me use an analogy. There is a spectrum of skill from being a novice reporter on regional radio to being Jeremy Paxman. What is it that Paxman does that the novice doesn't do? It is silly to expect the novice reporter to turn up and be Paxman on his or her first day of work, but with practice and experience, you can reasonably expect the novice to improve. Some novices want to be good enough for regional radio, some aim higher. In much the same fashion, there is a graduation in skill level from GP trainee to an experienced and competent GP.

Some trainee GPs want to pass, whereas others, even at this early stage in their career, want to refine their craft. If you are looking to really hone your craft, then it is useful to break each skill (active listening, negotiation, patient-centred management, etc.) into components, practise, and compare your performance to a model performance.

For those who simply want to get through the exam unscathed, my advice is to do a few of the cases from Part I and to look for patterns. Which aspects of the consultation do you regularly miss or do differently to the model? For instance, are you consistently not providing a brief explanation of the diagnosis before offering management options? Tackle those aspects of your consulting first and improve in broad brush strokes.

Part II

The cases in the second half assume a certain level of knowledge and skill and so provide less detail to role-players and candidates. The cases are not designed to teach specific skills in the same way as the first half of the book. Rather, the cases provide an opportunity to practise and revise, preferably with a group of peers so that the learning and feedback is provided by the group. For those cramming in the last few weeks, these cases are essential.

We hope that you enjoy the book and find your own way to work through the cases, improve your skills, and pass the exam!

Prashini Naidoo and Sonali Bapat
November 2015

Acknowledgements

Thank you to Dr Samantha Wild, my very dear friend, for her helpful comments and critiques over coffee and cake.

Thank you to the DMS Trainers, with whom I meet annually. You tease me about the articulate and magnificent Springboks, but I like you anyway, even Roland, the cider drinker and Martin, the limerick writer.

Finally, a reminder to my husband Anton – we may have flirted with a dairy herd and poly-tunnels in Wakkerstroom, but you still owe me a piggery at the foot of the Drakensberg Mountains.

Dedication

This book is dedicated to Suri and Lara who remind me to trust in tomorrow.

P.N.

Abbreviations

A&E	Accident and emergency department	DN	District Nurse
AA	Alcoholics Anonymous	DoH	Department of Health
ACR	Albumin–creatinine ratio	DSH	Deliberate self-harm
AF	Atrial fibrillation	DVLA	Driver and Vehicle Licensing Agency
AIDS	Acquired immune deficiency syndrome	DVT	Deep vein thrombosis
ALT	Alanine transaminase	ECG	Electrocardiogram
ARB	Angiotensin receptor blocker	ENT	Ear, nose and throat
AV	Atrioventricular	ESR	Erythrocyte sedimentation rate
BCC	Basal cell carcinoma	FBC	Full blood count
BD	Twice a day	FH	Familial hypercholesterolaemia
BG	Blood glucose	GA	General anaesthetic
BMI	Body mass index	GFR	Glomerular filtration rate
BP	Blood pressure	GI	Gastrointestinal
BPE	Benign prostatic enlargement	GMC	General Medical Council
bpm	Beats per minute	GORD	Gastro-oesophageal reflux disease
CBT	Cognitive behavioural therapy	Hb	Haemoglobin
CHC	Combined hormonal contraceptive	HBV	Hepatitis B virus
CKD	Chronic kidney disease	hCG	Human chorionic gonadotrophin
CMH	Community Mental Health	HDL	High-density lipoprotein
CNS	Central nervous system	HIV	Human immunodeficiency virus
COC	Combined oral contraceptive	HMB	Heavy menstrual bleeding
COPD	Chronic obstructive pulmonary disease	HRT	Hormone replacement therapy
CRP	C-reactive protein	HS	Heart sounds
CSA	Clinical skills assessment	HV	Health visitor
CTS	Carpal tunnel syndrome	IBD	Inflammatory bowel disease
CVS	Cardiovascular system	IBS	Irritable bowel syndrome
CXR	Chest X-ray	ICSI	Intracytoplasmic sperm injection
D&V	Diarrhoea and vomiting	IHD	Ischaemic heart disease
DEXA	Dual-energy X-ray absorptiometry	IM	Intramuscular
		IUD	Intrauterine device (e.g. copper coil)
		IUS	Intrauterine system (e.g. Mirena)

IV	Intravenous		PRN	As required
IVF	*In vitro* fertilisation		PSA	Prostate-specific antigen
LDL	Low-density lipoprotein		PT	Prothrombin time
LFTs	Liver function tests		PV	*per vagina*
LMP	Last menstrual period		QDS	Four times a day
LUTI	Lower urinary tract infection		RCT	Randomised controlled trial
LUTS	Lower urinary tract symptoms		RS	Respiratory system
MC&S	Microscopy, culture and sensitivities		SARS	Sudden acute respiratory syndrome
MCH	Mean cell haemoglobin		SGPT	Serum glutamic-pyruvic transaminase
MCV	Mean corpuscular volume			
MDU	Medical Defence Union		SHBG	Sex hormone binding globulin
MI	Myocardial infarction		SIGN	Scottish Intercollegiate Guidelines Network
MS	Multiple sclerosis			
MSU	Mid-stream urine		SLE	Systemic lupus erythematosus
MT	Metatarsal		SSRI	Selective serotonin reuptake inhibitor
MTP	Metatarsophalangeal			
NAD	No abnormality detected		STD	Sexually transmitted disease
NAI	Non-accidental injury		STI	Sexually transmitted infection
NICE	National Institute for Health and Care Excellence		SVT	Supraventricular tachycardia
			TCA	Tricyclic antidepressant
NSAID	Non-steroidal anti-inflammatory drug		TDS	Three times a day
			TFTs	Thyroid function tests
NVD	Normal vaginal delivery		TIA	Transient ischaemic attack
OAB	Overactive bladder		TOP	Termination of pregnancy
OCD	Obsessive compulsive disorder		TPO	Thyroid peroxidase
OD	Once a day		TSH	Thyroid-stimulating hormone
OPD	Out-patient department		U&Es	Urea and electrolytes
OTC	Over-the-counter		UC	Ulcerative colitis
O/E	On examination		UKMEC	UK Medical Eligibility Criteria
PCOS	Polycystic ovary syndrome		URTI	Upper respiratory tract infection
PE	Pulmonary embolism		USS	Ultrasound scan
PF	Plantar fasciitis		UTI	Urinary tract infection
POP	Progesterone-only contraceptive pill		VT	Ventricular tachycardia
PR	*per rectum*		WBC	White blood count

CASE 1 Muslim diabetic

INFORMATION FOR THE DOCTOR

Name	Fazeela Amir
Age	52
Social and family history	Married, two adult children
Past medical history	• NIDDM diagnosed 2 years ago • Hypertension for 5 years • Mild eczema
Current medication	• Ramipril 10mg daily • Metformin 850mg BD • Gliclazide 80mg BD • Atorvastatin 20mg OD
Blood tests HbA1c Plasma fasting glucose Fasting cholesterol Fasting HDL cholesterol TSH Alkaline phosphatase Total bilirubin Albumin Creatinine level U&Es BMI BP	*Blood tests done 2 months ago* 6.8g% 6.5mmol/L (3.65–5.5) 4.2mmol/L 0.9mmol/L (0.8–1.8) 1.95 (0.35–5.5) 263IU/L (95–280) 14µmol/L (3–17) 46g/L (35–50) 99µmol/L (70–150) within the normal range 28 131/86

INFORMATION FOR THE PATIENT

You are Fazeela Amir, a 52-year-old primary school teaching assistant. You have come to see the doctor to discuss your diabetic medication over Ramadan. You started taking gliclazide earlier this year. The follow-up blood tests showed that it was controlling your blood sugars well. A friend told you that the dose of your medication may need to be changed over Ramadan, so you've come to see the doctor for advice.

You are a devout Muslim. You observe Ramadan and fast from sunrise to sunset – during this time you will not eat food or take any fluids. You have not fasted when you were pregnant, but made the days up later in the year.

You have changed the type of food you cook. You used to cook food with higher fat and sugar but since your diabetes and your husband's cholesterol problems, you use less oil and less sugar. You have started to use more nuts, low calorie sweeteners and fruit in your baking.

You do gentle exercise, usually a 30 minute walk every day. You'd like to continue with your walking and think that it may be best to do the walking after the evening meal (iftar).

You present to the doctor expecting to discuss the changes you should make to your medication over Ramadan. It has not occurred to you not to fast.

Information to reveal if asked

General information about yourself:

- You work as a primary school teaching assistant. You enjoy the work. It is not a physically demanding job.
- You tend to cook most of your meals from scratch. You occasionally eat out. Over Ramadan, you intend to eat at home. Either you or a family member will do the cooking.
- You eat meat and vegetables. You prefer savoury fried snacks and your husband has a sweet tooth. However, Ramadan for you is about abstention and sacrifice, so you tend to cook plain and wholesome food over this period.
- You have never smoked tobacco and do not drink alcohol.

Further details about your condition:

- You have been diabetic for five years, initially diet controlled. Last year, you took your metformin as usual and continued with your fast.

- One of the Muslim teachers at the school said she didn't know if you could take your medication and still fast; her father had to change his insulin injections at Ramadan.

Your ideas:

- You do not see your diabetes as an illness that prevents you from fasting. You also don't see how fasting could be damaging to your health. You think that you make too little hormone to move the sugar you eat around your body, so if you fast, you have less sugar which is better for your health.

- Most of the diabetic Muslims you know fast. The only ones who do not fast are people who are very sick, pregnant or in hospital.

- Over the years, you have tended to maintain your weight during Ramadan. Your husband loses a bit of weight but he soon puts it on after the fast with Eid.

- You are prepared to take tablets with the morning and evening meal; luckily nothing is needed during the fasting hours. You want to continue with your exercise.

- You do not like testing your blood sugars. If asked to test blood glucose regularly, you seem a bit daunted. You are not sure if this is allowed during the fast.

Your concerns:

- You are worried about being advised against fasting. You are worried that the doctor may not understand your religious beliefs nor recognise how important this is to you.

Your expectations:

- You expect to get information about whether you need to change your diabetes medication over the fast.

Medical history

- You consider yourself to be healthy. You do not currently have any side-effects from your current medication.

Social history

- You are happily married. One child is at University studying psychology and one is working overseas.

- You enjoy your current social life.

Information to reveal if examined

If the doctor asks to do your blood pressure, hand him/her a card saying "BP 130/80".

SUGGESTED APPROACH TO THE CONSULTATION

Targeted history taking:

- Obtain details of the fast. When and what will she eat? When and how much will she drink? What exercise will she undertake?

- How does she normally take her medication?

- How does she see her diabetes affecting or being affected by the fast (her ideas)?

- How well controlled is Fazeela's diabetes? It is important to stratify Fazeela's risk over Ramadan into high, moderate or low risk. Has she had any hypoglycaemic episodes, especially in the last three months? Does she have any acute illness? Is she prone to catching minor illness at work? Does she do heavy physical activity with her job or in her leisure time?

- What are her concerns? Is she worried about the dose and timing of medication over Ramadan? Is she worried about doing more blood sugar monitoring?

- What are her expectations? Does she expect specific dietary and exercise advice; medication changes; referral to Diabetes specialist clinics or follow-up bloods after Ramadan?

- Is she prepared to change her medication?

Targeted examination:

- This case does not require the candidate to perform a targeted physical examination.

Clinical management:

- Having stratified her into a moderate risk category (she is on a sulphonylurea), build on her existing idea that she is perfectly capable of fasting but there are certain times when it is important to be sensible and not fast, such as if she becomes unwell with an acute illness, or develops symptoms of dehydration, hypo- or hyperglycaemia.

- Discuss the timing and size of meals. If she is having a smaller meal (one-third of her calories) before sunrise and a larger meal (two-thirds of her calories) after sunset, then she could continue metformin 850mg bd, atorvastatin 20mg at night but reduce gliclazide to 40mg in the morning and stay on gliclazide 80mg at night.

- Despite the reduced dose of sulphonylurea, if her BG drops below 3.9 or goes above 16.7mmol/L, you would advise her to break her fast. The chances of such swings in BG are further reduced by following a healthy diet. Reassure her that BG monitoring during fasting is not considered as breaking one's fast. BG need only be undertaken if she suspects a low glucose or feels unwell.

- Discuss diet: she intends to have a 'wholesome' diet, which is entirely appropriate. Complex carbohydrates (beans, rice, lentils) and high fibre foods (wholegrain bread, vegetables, salads, nuts, dates) should be baked or grilled rather than cooked with saturated fats, or if shallow frying or making curry, use olive oil rather than ghee. She is quite correct to avoid Indian sweets (mithai). It may be better to avoid coffee which encourages diuresis and hydrate with other fluids instead.

- Discuss exercise: doing 30 minutes of walking after the larger evening meal is entirely appropriate.

- Address the patient's concerns about being advised not to fast. Fazeela is being proactive and seeking advice early. If she puts small changes in place, her risk of being unwell during Ramadan is reduced. However, if she does become unwell despite her best efforts, especially if BG is <3.9 or >16.7mmol/L, then she should really consider breaking her fast and perhaps do the missed fast days later in the year.

- Address the patient's expectations about medication changes.

- Arrange follow-up, possibly with a repeat HbA1c after Ramadan, to change medication doses back to usual regimes.

Interpersonal skills:

This case tests the doctor's ability to respond sensitively to a patient's request to a change in her diabetic treatment for religious reasons.

Good communication with the patient:

- is sensitive to her beliefs and values.

- explores what the patient wants to achieve and gives tailored advice to help her reach these goals safely.

- involves discussing how to take medication during Ramadan, how to monitor for problems and what to do if problems arise.

Poor communication with the patient:

- makes the patient feel that her beliefs and values are being dismissed without consideration; the doctor seems motivated by his or her own strongly held beliefs.

- recites the advice in a protocol-driven manner; there is little to and fro discussion; the doctor is not seen to build on ideas the patient has offered. Most of the talking, especially in the second half of the consultation, is being done by the doctor.

- displays little or no curiosity in the patient as a person.

BACKGROUND KNOWLEDGE REQUIRED FOR THIS CASE

Gilani, A (2011) **Ramadan and your diabetic patient**. NHS, Greater Glasgow and Clyde.

http://library.nhsggc.org.uk/mediaAssets/My%20HSD/2011-05-31-RAMADAN_RESOURCE_PACK.pdf

Those who are considered Islamically exempt from fasting are:

- the frail and elderly
- children
- those who have a chronic condition whereby participating in fasting would be detrimental to their health
- those who cannot understand the purpose of fasting, i.e. those who have learning difficulties or those who suffer from severe mental health problems
- travellers (those travelling greater than 50 miles)*
- those acutely unwell*
- pregnant and breast-feeding women*

*Considered to be temporarily exempt. Fasts must be made up at a later date but if unable to do so then fidyah must be given (fidyah is when those who are considered exempt and do not fast can compensate by giving alms to the poor).

Relevant literature

For an excellent flow chart on how to manage medication, see:

http://sitelife.bmj.com/ver1.0//Content/images/store/13/3/ad981831-14f2-4c9f-b34b-60f6b6544a57.Full.jpg

CASE 2 PCOS

INFORMATION FOR THE DOCTOR

Name	Christina Whittaker
Age	42
Social and family history	Married, one teenage child
Past medical history	• Abdominal pain 4 days ago – admitted overnight to hospital but discharge summary is not available as yet • Migraine 7 years ago • PCOS 15 years ago
Current medication	Co-codamol 30/500 – 2t QDS
Blood tests Liver function tests Renal function tests FBC and ESR Random glucose Serum cholesterol HDL Fasting triglyceride TSH Random glucose Cervical smear BMI BP	*Blood tests done 4 days ago* within normal range within normal range within normal range 6.9mmol/L (3.0–5.5 for fasting glucose) 6.1mmol/L (3.65–6.5) 1.0mmol/L (0.8–1.8) 1.9mmol/L (0.55–1.9) *Blood tests from 2 years ago* within normal range 5.8mmol/L (3.0–5.5) *From smear consultation 1 year ago* Normal – recall in 3 years 28.3 134/82

INFORMATION FOR THE PATIENT

You are Christina Whittaker, a 42-year-old Operating Department Practitioner (ODP), who has come to get a sick note for work.

You saw a GP 4 days ago and were sent to the hospital with an acute abdomen. The ultrasound scan did not show an inflamed appendix; the internal scan showed free fluid and a thickened womb lining. You went on to have a CT scan which showed a small cyst on your adrenal gland, which you were told was an incidental finding but will require a follow-up MRI, for which an appointment will be posted to you. The hospital doctors suspect that you had a ruptured ovarian cyst. They sent you home on analgesia, and said they would send you an appointment for Gynae outpatients to discuss the thickened womb lining and ovarian cysts. You had PCOS in the past, for which you had taken metformin but your symptoms improved and you stopped metformin 4 years ago.

As an ODP, you have some background medical knowledge. You suspect that the PCOS has become symptomatic and one of the cysts ruptured, giving you the severe pain 4 days ago. The pain has eased considerably. You are taking paracetamol during the day, co-codamol at night, regular diclofenac which the hospital supplied, to good effect and without side-effects. You want the GP today to sign you off work for a week. You don't think you can make good decisions while on the medication and you need a bit of time to recover before returning to Orthopaedic theatre work.

You would also like to restart metformin. You used metformin for PCOS for a few years. You don't remember having side-effects. One day you stopped taking it; your symptoms did not recur, so you stayed off the medication and you didn't mind the irregular light periods. You did not get on with the combined pill: you developed migraine, mood swings and put on weight. Your family is complete; you husband has had a vasectomy.

You present to the doctor wishing to discuss your PCOS. Your opening statement is *"So, it looks like my polycystic ovaries are playing up again".*

Information to reveal if asked

General information about yourself:

- You work at the district general hospital as an ODP.
- You really enjoy your work and feel that as a hospital employee, the consultants treating you there are giving you personalised care.
- Your teenage son and your husband were slightly shocked by your hospital admission, but you only stayed in for one night. Your husband has returned to work.

Further details about your condition:

- If specifically asked, you have never suffered from acne, greasy skin or hirsutism. You have had irregular periods – they tend to be light, lasting only 3–4 days and occurring every 6–8 weeks. You also have difficulty losing weight. You did not have difficulty getting pregnant. You had an uneventful pregnancy. The original diagnosis of PCOS was made on a scan and because you had such irregular periods. You don't remember there being a problem with your blood tests.

- You are an only child. You do not have a family history of PCOS. Your dad has hypertension.

- You do not want to take hormones. You think that you are too old and too overweight to take the Pill. You prefer to take metformin. It worked well for you. You think you ran out of tablets one day and you were supposed to make an appointment to get a repeat prescription but something happened, and before you knew it, 2 months had passed. You felt well during those 2 months and thought that maybe you didn't need treatment with metformin any longer.

Your ideas:

- You think that your acute abdomen could have been a ruptured ovarian cyst because of your PCOS and the free fluid found on the ultrasound scan. You are a little bit worried about the small cyst that the CT discovered on your adrenal gland, but you read up about adrenal cysts on the internet and found that most cysts are benign and even if they are malignant, they tend to be non-functioning adenomas. You also read that a follow-up MRI, which the hospital is scheduling, is a good investigation.

- You have been referred to Gynae to discuss the 'thickened' womb lining. You intend to keep this appointment but if this is all due to PCOS, you'd like to go back on your metformin now.

Your concerns:

- You are worried that the Gynae outpatient appointment may take a few weeks to come through and you'd rather not have another ruptured ovarian cyst while waiting, so you'd like the GP to start the metformin today.

Your expectations:

- You expect a sick note for work and a prescription for metformin.

Medical history

You are in good general health, and are not on long-term medication. You get the occasional migraine, usually stress-related, but taking paracetamol, ibuprofen and lying down tend to help to resolve the attack.

Social history

You are happily married.

You are one of the senior ODPs and you instruct trainee ODPs during their placements in orthopaedic theatre.

Information to reveal if examined

Abdominal examination – soft and slightly tender R lower quadrant.

If the doctor asks to weigh you, hand him/her a card saying "BMI 28".

SUGGESTED APPROACH TO THE CONSULTATION

Targeted history taking:

- What are Christina's symptoms now?

- What is her understanding of her recent illness and the hospital's management plan?

- What are her concerns? Is she worried about the adrenal cyst, the thickened womb lining, the risk of another ovarian cyst rupture?

- What are her expectations: does she want you to interpret the radiology findings for her, obtain a copy of the discharge summary, coordinate her care, order any outstanding investigations, provide a sick note, treat the PCOS prior to her Gynae appointment?

- How was her PCOS originally diagnosed? What are her current symptoms? What are her treatment options?

- What does she already know about PCOS and lifestyle changes (losing weight; reducing carbohydrates and increasing physical activity) to improve insulin resistance?

- Does she have contra-indications to co-cyprindiol or combined hormonal contraception (CHC)?

Targeted examination:

- A targeted examination is not required in this case.

Clinical management:

- Discuss the data that Christina has presented. Do you have sufficient data, in the absence of a hospital discharge summary, to make a decision about a sick note and prescribing metformin?

- Discuss your decisions with Christina and negotiate a shared management plan. If you prescribe, discuss dose, side-effects and follow-up. If you decide not to prescribe, Christina is unhappy so be prepared to defend your decision and get Christina to buy in to your delayed prescription.

- Discuss the importance of a healthy lifestyle – weight loss and exercise improve insulin resistance, increase ovulation and reduce cardiovascular risk.

- Offer Christina annual BMI, BP and diabetes screening.

- Address the patient's idea that metformin needs to be started as soon as possible to prevent ovarian cyst formation and other complications of PCOS. Metformin has been found to be less effective than Dianette at improving menstrual regularity. We don't know if metformin prevents type 2 diabetes, reduces cardiovascular events or prevents endometrial cancer in women with

PCOS. However, compared to Dianette, metformin has a lower incidence of precipitating weight gain, raising BP or aggravating headaches. It is important to discuss the risks and benefits of metformin. Christina is 42 and suffers migraine, hence Dianette and CHC are contra-indicated.

- Also discuss non-drug treatments – a low calorie, low glycaemic index diet combined with exercise can reduce PCOS symptoms and CV risk.

- Address the patient's concerns about ovarian cyst recurrence and developing PCOS complications.

- Address the patient's expectations of a sick note and treatment for PCOS. Once all the treatment options for PCOS have been explained and the low risk of ovarian cyst complications discussed, the patient's urgency for a prescription may have decreased and she may want further written information or some time to think options through before making a final decision.

- Confirm Christina's understanding of PCOS, its treatment options, its link with insulin resistance and the need for screening for associated CV risk factors on a regular basis.

- Arrange a follow-up appointment.

Interpersonal skills:

This case tests the doctor's ability to communicate with a patient who is also a health professional. It also tests the doctor's ability to use the available (incomplete) data to make decisions. There is some uncertainty (the doctor does not have access to the scan results at the time of consultation). How the doctor behaves in the face of uncertainty is tested.

Good communication with the patient:

- explores what the patient already knows and understands about her health and uses this information to decide if he or she has acquired sufficient data (in the absence of scan reports or a discharge summary) to make prescribing decisions.

- empathises with the patient's fear of developing further PCOS complications, but puts this risk in perspective.

- discusses the pros and cons of various treatment options, thereby revealing an evidence-based approach to treatment.

- explains the global picture of increased CV risk to the patient and arranges long-term screening.

Poor communication with the patient:

- does not gather data systematically from the patient. The doctor could be overly hasty in prescribing. Alternatively, the doctor seems, from the off, completely unprepared to accept any uncertainty and refuses to prescribe without first listening to the patient's story.

- does not address the patient's expectations but veers into a discussion about issues that do not currently concern the patient, such as the adrenal cyst. If the doctor discusses the possibility of a testosterone-producing adrenal cyst, how does he or she break the news and cope with the patient's anguish? What tests does he or she order?
- does not provide sufficient information about the pros and cons of the treatment options to enable the patient to make an informed decision.

BACKGROUND KNOWLEDGE REQUIRED FOR THIS CASE

NICE (Feb 2013) **Polycystic ovary syndrome: metformin in women not planning pregnancy**. www.nice.org.uk/advice/esuom6

Metformin is licensed in the UK for the control of blood glucose in people with type 2 diabetes. It has also been used to treat polycystic ovary syndrome (PCOS). Metformin is not licensed in the UK for this indication so its use in PCOS is off-label.

The NICE Feb 2013 guidance is based on a review of five small randomised controlled trials (RCTs) included in a Cochrane systematic review, and four RCTs published after the Cochrane review. They summarise:

1. Hirsutism: there is no good evidence that regimens containing metformin are statistically significantly different from co-cyprindiol in controlling hirsutism in women with PCOS.
2. Acne: two small studies found no statistically significant difference between metformin and co-cyprindiol in effects on acne but the assessment methods were unclear.
3. Periods: metformin was less effective at improving menstrual regularity than co-cyprindiol.
4. Long-term risk: there was no or insufficient data in the studies included in this evidence summary from which to draw conclusions on the effectiveness of metformin for long-term outcomes such as preventing type 2 diabetes, CV events or endometrial cancer in women with PCOS.

Disadvantages of metformin: it is associated with gastrointestinal adverse effects (nausea, vomiting and diarrhoea), which can be severe. The Cochrane review found that metformin caused a significantly higher incidence of gastrointestinal adverse effects that were severe (leading to treatment discontinuation) compared with co-cyprindiol.

Advantages: metformin had a significantly lower incidence of other severe adverse effects (weight gain, high blood pressure, depression, chest pain and headache). Among all nine trials there was significant heterogeneity in the rates of treatment discontinuation, which was not always because of adverse effects.

The annual cost of metformin at 1.5–2g per day ranges from £30.03 to £83.20, depending on whether standard or modified-release tablets are prescribed.

Alternative commonly used treatments for hirsutism, acne and menstrual irregularity in PCOS in women not planning pregnancy are:

1. Co-cyprindiol, a combination product containing cyproterone and ethinylestradiol. Co-cyprindiol is licensed for treating severe acne refractory to prolonged oral antibiotic therapy, and moderately severe hirsutism. It is not licensed specifically for use in PCOS.
2. The combined oral contraceptive pill. This is not licensed for controlling menstrual irregularity in PCOS.

Relevant literature

For a good patient information sheet, see www.rcog.org.uk/globalassets/documents/patients/patient-information-leaflets/gynaecology/polycystic-ovary-syndrome-pcos.pdf

CASE 3 Alcoholic

INFORMATION FOR THE DOCTOR

Name	Adam James
Age	29
Social and family history	Separated, one child aged 3 who lives with mum
Past medical history	• Alcohol problem drinking • Low mood • Was on risk register 2 years ago and was known to social services and health visitor

The medical record of his **last consultation** in surgery 2 weeks ago reads:

"Described AA as a waste of time and finds it difficult to commit to sessions – has to work shifts. Says he did not drink for 10 days, then went out with mates and drank heavily. Was late next day collecting his son; delayed on 3 hour road trip. Wife was angry and they had a row. Drove back without spending time with son. Sertraline helped low mood but ran out of tablets 5 days ago before he could get to surgery today. Sleep is still a problem. Plan: try zopiclone 7.5mg over next 2 weeks, then review."

Current medication	Zopiclone 7.5mg once nightly, as needed
Blood tests Full blood count Liver function tests	*Blood tests done 2 months ago* normal normal
BP	134/84

INFORMATION FOR THE PATIENT

You are Adam James, a 29-year-old chef, who has come to discuss the problems you experience with sleep. The doctor you saw 2 weeks ago thought sleeping tablets might help. The tablets she prescribed help you to fall asleep but you still wake up after 3 hours and you have difficulty getting off to sleep again. You toss and turn in the night. You are tired in the mornings and your concentration during the day is reduced. You don't have the energy to follow things through and you forget about things. For example, you forgot to arrange a GP appointment to get more anti-depressant medication, so you ran out of medication completely. The last doctor was cross. She said these drugs can't just be stopped and started on a whim, so she said it would best not to prescribe them. Another example of not seeing things through was when you forgot to book your car in for a MOT, and you couldn't tax it in time. You had to call your wife to ask if she'd drive your son to you. That led to further arguments.

You have had sleep problems for many years. You started to drink more alcohol to get off to sleep and to stop you from thinking about your bad luck. A typical example of bad luck occurred at a recent night out with a work colleague. You asked a drunken man to stop hitting on a woman, he swung, a fight broke out and all of you were thrown out. In the process you lost your keys. You had to have the locks replaced at a time when you could not afford the additional expense. Everyone tells you that you drink too much. If you could sleep better, without alcohol, and not feel as if you had the world's worst luck, then you'd cut down on your drinking.

You present to the doctor expecting to be fobbed off with more advice about cutting down the alcohol but you would really like some help, specifically medication, for the sleep difficulties. Your opening statement is *"I think I might need some stronger sleeping tablets doc"*.

Information to reveal if asked

General information about yourself:

- You are a chef at a local hotel. You believe that you are good at your job. A few years ago, you won a regional competition, but your career has slowed a bit with your separation and financial problems.

- You can be asked to work the breakfast and lunch service, or the evening service. You prefer the evening service but the choice is not always up to you.

- During an argument with your wife, you threw a beer can. It hit the wall and ricocheted, hitting her on the face. Your young son witnessed this. She reported it as domestic violence and social services were involved. She moved out and is living near her family. You want to maintain contact with your son.

Further details about your condition:

- If specifically asked about your drinking, you discuss how for the last 2 months, you have cut down your drinking from 4–6 cans of beer every day after work to 2 beers per night and none on the weekends when you see your son.

- You have never taken recreational drugs.

- Your father had problems with alcohol which contributed to your parents' divorce. Your mum told you that he died of pneumonia because he wouldn't seek help, preferring to stay at home and ignore his symptoms.

- If asked, you feel anxious about coming to the doctor. You feel on edge a lot of the time and find it hard to relax. You worry about what people think. Right now, you are worried the doctor thinks you are a time-waster, but you are also worried about your bad sleep. At the same time as being worried, you are also angry with everybody – with the doctors for not helping you, with your wife's behaviour, with work who change your shifts at short notice. Little things like someone whistling in the kitchen annoy you massively. You get irritated so easily and you worry about embarrassing yourself or being laughed at to the extent that you avoid a lot of social situations. You prefer to go back to an empty flat even though you know you just lie there waiting for sleep that won't come.

Your ideas:

- You think that you can control your drinking but you need help with the sleep. You think you worry too much and can't relax.

Your concerns:

- You are worried that you are turning into your father and, if things continue, you will become increasingly isolated. You worry that if you can't sort out the sleeping, you will self-medicate with alcohol.

Your expectations:

- You expect to be fobbed off but you are prepared to stand your ground and get some help with the sleep problem.

Medical history

Physically, you are in good general health, and do not have any tremors, shakes or sweating.

Social history

You are separated. You are not in a relationship. You prefer to talk to one or two people. You get uncomfortable in groups. You feel self-conscious and think people are judging you.

Information to reveal if examined

An examination is not required.

SUGGESTED APPROACH TO THE CONSULTATION

Targeted history taking:

- Take a detailed history of Adam's sleep: when does he go to bed; wake up; how long does it take him to fall asleep; how often does he wake up; how long does he stay awake for; how does he feel during the day; does he nap; how much alcohol/caffeine does he drink; what is the timing of his meal/exercise relative to his sleep; self-rate the quality of his sleep.

- Explore Adam's ideas about why his sleep may be poor. Ask him to describe his worries. What types of thoughts go around in his head preventing him from relaxing? Does he worry at other times? How would he describe his mood on most days? How does he feel at the moment? How does he feel at work? How does he feel when doing something he enjoys? How does he feel in groups?

- What are his concerns? Explore his family history and his fears.

- He stated his expectations at the outset. Having used 2 weeks of zopiclone at the higher dose, you are limited in your prescribing options. NICE advises the use of the lowest effective dose of hypnotic for the shortest period possible, usually for 2–4 weeks, with re-assessment after 2 weeks.

- Are there any other reasons for the disturbed sleep? Take a good alcohol history.

- Did he feel anxious, on edge, or irritable before he started drinking or did the feelings trigger or exacerbate the drinking?

Targeted examination:

- Perform a brief mental state examination for anxiety.

Clinical management:

- Summarise for him his feelings, thoughts and behaviours. *"So, to summarise, you describe how you feel anxious, irritable, and jittery in a lot of situations. You think that you will embarrass yourself and people will laugh at you. You avoid socialising, especially in groups, and drink to feel more relaxed."*

- Discuss a possible diagnosis of social anxiety disorder.

- Reassure Adam that the sleep problem and alcohol are symptoms of the underlying anxiety, a condition that is treatable. Discuss the treatment options and consider signposting to suitable patient information leaflets.

- Address Adam's ideas: that 'stronger' tablets or alcohol are needed to attain good sleep. CBT is first-line treatment, but if declined, drug therapy may be offered. SSRIs (such as sertraline) for the treatment of anxiety are very likely to help with the sleep, but it may take several weeks before the quantity and quality of sleep improve. Tricyclics are not a good first or second choice.

- Address the patient's concerns about turning into an alcoholic recluse. *"If you didn't treat your anxiety and continued to drink, what could happen? If you treated your anxiety and did not rely on alcohol, what would happen? On a scale of 1–5, how motivated are you to get this treated and to stick to the treatment? What help do you need in committing to treatment?"*

- Address the patient's expectations for help with a difficult problem, but resist the temptation to prescribe inappropriately. Sedative drugs (such as sedating antidepressants, antihistamines, chloral hydrate, clomethiazole, and barbiturates) are not recommended for the management of insomnia; hypnotics may be used.

- Confirm his understanding of social anxiety disorder and provide sufficient information about the treatment options with CBT, CBT-based self-help and/or SSRIs, to enable him to decide on treatment.

- Arrange suitable follow-up and/or referral.

Interpersonal skills:

This case tests the doctor's ability to keep an open mind and explore a presenting problem more deeply, resulting in a new diagnosis. It also tests the doctor's ability to remain optimistic and supportive in the face of irritability, apathy (loss of motivation) and anger.

Good communication with the patient:

- encourages the patient to tell his story through the skilful use of open questions: *"Tell me more about your sleep/your feelings/your thoughts when you are lying in bed/about what the alcohol does for you?"*

- makes statements that help to build the patient's confidence: *"I am really impressed by the way you came back to the surgery, feeling the way you did, to tackle this problem head-on."*

- builds trust through reflective listening: *"It sounds like…"*

- summarises well: *"Let me see if I understand so far…"*

- encourages change: *"On a scale of 0–5, how motivated are you to change?"*

Poor communication with the patient:

- makes assumptions about the patient's drinking, sleep, motivation for seeking help.

- prejudges and dismisses the patient.

- fails to develop a therapeutic alliance with the patient.

- is prescriptive in his or her management.

BACKGROUND KNOWLEDGE REQUIRED FOR THIS CASE

Identification questions for anxiety disorders
GAD-2 scale

The GAD-2 screening tool consists of the first 2 questions of the GAD-7 scale:

Over the last 2 weeks, how often have you been bothered by the following problems:

1. Feeling nervous, anxious or on edge

2. Not being able to stop or control worrying

Score 0 for "not at all", 1 for "several days", 2 for "more than half the days, 3 for "nearly every day".

If the person scores less than 3 on the GAD-2 scale, but you are still concerned they may have an anxiety disorder, ask the following: *"Do you find yourself avoiding places or activities and does this cause you problems?"*

For the full GAD-7, see:

Spitzer RL, Kroenke K, Williams JB, *et al.* (2006) A brief measure for assessing generalized anxiety disorder: the GAD-7. *Arch. Intern. Med.* **166**: 1092–7.

NICE guidelines (2013) CG159: Social anxiety disorder. www.nice.org.uk/guidance/CG159

Obtain a detailed description of the person's current social anxiety and associated problems and circumstances including:

- feared and avoided social situations
- what they are afraid might happen in social situations (for example, looking anxious, blushing, sweating, trembling or appearing boring)
- anxiety symptoms
- view of self
- content of self-image
- safety-seeking behaviours
- focus of attention in social situations
- anticipatory and post-event processing
- occupational, educational, financial and social circumstances
- medication, alcohol and recreational drug use.

Relevant literature

For an introduction to motivational interviewing techniques, see
www.derby.ac.uk/files/motivational_interviewing.pdf

There are five methods that are useful throughout the process of motivational
interviewing.

1. Open questions
2. Affirmations
3. Reflective listening
4. Summarising
5. Eliciting change talk

The first four are used to explore ambivalence (uncertainty) and clarify reasons for
change. The fifth is more directive.

CASE 4 **Metabolic syndrome**

INFORMATION FOR THE DOCTOR

Name	Chris Johnson
Age	22
Social and family history	Single, no children
Past medical history	• Tonsillitis 3 years ago • Minor head injury 7 years ago
Current medication	Diclofenac 50mg thrice daily
Blood tests CRP Alkaline phosphatase Total bilirubin ALT* Plasma creatinine Plasma urate* Plasma albumin Alkaline phosphatase Total bilirubin ALT/SGPT* Plasma creatinine Plasma urate* Plasma albumin Fasting glucose Serum cholesterol HDL Fasting triglyceride* O/E height O/E weight BMI* BP	*Blood tests done last week* 8 (<8) 181IU/L (95–280) 6µmol/L (3–17) 66IU/L (10–45) 112µmol/L (70–150) 534µmol/L (210–480) 48g/L (35–50) *Blood tests from one year ago* 177IU/L (95–280) 12µmol/L (3–17) 92IU/L (10–45) 100µmol/L (70–150) 522µmol/L (210–480) 47g/L (35–50) 4.9 (3.0–5.5) 5.5 (3.65–6.5) 1.24 (0.8–1.8) 2.6 (0.55–1.9) 176cm 94kg 30.3 128/78

INFORMATION FOR THE PATIENT

You are Chris Johnson, a 22-year-old bank employee, who has come to discuss the blood results you had last week. You saw a doctor last week with a painful left foot. The doctor was not sure if you had gout so he requested some blood tests.

Since last week, the pain is much better, having improved from 8/10 to 1–2/10 once the anti-inflammatories kicked in. The left toe was painful at the MTP joint *(which you point to)*. What surprised the doctor last week was the lack of redness and swelling of the joint. The doctor told you that gout usually causes the skin to become red and shiny. While your joint was very tender to touch, it looked normal. You can now weight bear without difficulty, whereas last week, the pain had limited walking and any pressure put through the foot was agonising.

You found elevating the foot and using an ice-pack after work helped. The diclofenac also gave good relief, unlike the over-the-counter ibuprofen which you tried before you saw the doctor.

The doctor you saw last week wanted to check your bloods to see if your uric acid was raised. Also, the tests you had last year after the first episode of foot pain, which was also thought to be gout, had shown some liver problems. The doctor repeated other tests to see if the liver problem picked up on in last year's tests had persisted. You are a bit worried about these liver tests. You don't drink a huge amount of alcohol. Last year you were advised to cut down on your drinking, which you did. You also increased your daily activity; you now walk to work, weather permitting. You try to eat fewer pre-prepared meals but cooking is not something you enjoy.

You present to the doctor expecting to be told that your blood tests show gout. Your opening statement is *"So, do my blood tests show gout doctor?"*.

Information to reveal if asked

General information about yourself:

- You work at a local bank.
- Last week, a colleague gave you a ride to work and you were able to continue with your sedentary job.
- You are fixing up the house you bought, but had to put the DIY on hold.

Further details about your condition:

- If specifically asked about your lifestyle, you discuss how since last year, you cut down your drinking from 5 to 8 beers three times per week to 5 beers per night on Fridays and Saturdays. The drinking increases during rugby season.

- You have never taken recreational drugs, you have not travelled recently and you have not had unprotected sex.

- You had a tattoo at a reputable parlour four years ago.

- You have not experienced excessive thirst, excessive urination, nor do you wake up at night to pass urine.

- You feel well in yourself and do not have digestive complaints.

Your ideas:

- You think that your symptoms are due to gout, but feel you are a bit young to have developed gout. Could the foot pain be something else?

- You don't think you drink very heavily compared to your rugby mates, so you are puzzled by the abnormal liver tests.

Your concerns:

- You are worried that other causes of foot pain may have been overlooked. Should you get an X-ray of your foot?

Your expectations:

- You expect to get information about the blood tests.

Medical history

You are in good general health, and are not on long-term medication. You have not used protein supplements or 'steroids' to build muscle.

Social history

You have a girlfriend.

You enjoy being part of the rugby club and play tighthead prop.

Information to reveal if examined

Abdominal examination – no masses palpable; soft and non-tender.

If the doctor asks to weigh you, hand him/her a card saying "BMI 32".

If the doctor asks to measure your waist circumference, hand over a card saying "central obesity".

SUGGESTED APPROACH TO THE CONSULTATION

Targeted history taking:

- What are Chris's symptoms now?
- What are his ideas about why the blood tests were taken and what did he make of last year's results?
- What are his concerns? Is he worried that he might be asked to give up alcohol?
- What are his expectations? It is obvious from his opening statement that he wants an explanation of last week's test results; however, is he aware of the link between gout and liver problems?
- Are there any other reasons for abnormal liver function tests – alcohol, drugs, foreign travel, unprotected sexual intercourse, diabetes, family history?
- What does he already know about fatty liver and the lifestyle changes (losing weight and increasing physical activity) required?
- How much of a verbal or written explanation does he require?

Targeted examination:

- Ask to perform a brief, targeted abdominal examination, and elicit BMI and waist circumference.

Clinical management:

- Discuss the blood results and examination findings: he has a raised ALT, serum urate, triglycerides and central obesity, all of which possibly suggest fatty liver with or without metabolic syndrome.
- Discuss what should be done about the raised ALT: he needs to stop alcohol completely and recheck his LFTs in four to six weeks. If the ALT remains high, then further blood tests (viral serology, ferritin, prothrombin time) and an ultrasound scan may be needed.
- Reassure Chris that, in the early stages, the liver recovers well if a healthier lifestyle is adopted.
- Negotiate goals for Chris to work towards and ask him what help he may need in reaching these goals. Consider food diaries and review with the practice nurse for healthy eating advice.
- Address the patient's ideas: that eating too much meat causes gout. A low protein diet is less important than a healthy, balanced diet. Discuss the importance of a low calorie diet rich in dietary fibre, with unsaturated fats, carbohydrates with a low glycaemic index and plenty of fresh fruit, i.e. a 'Mediterranean diet'.

- Address the patient's concerns about being told to eat less pre-prepared food and being advised to cook from scratch. Cutting out snacks, eating more fruit, drinking <21 units per week and exercising for 45 minutes would be an excellent start.

- Address the patient's expectations that an X-ray be done: an X-ray may be useful if the diagnosis of gout is in doubt. Two blood tests have already confirmed a marginally raised serum urate; sepsis or rheumatoid arthritis is not suspected.

- Confirm his understanding of gout, its treatment with anti-inflammatories, its link with metabolic syndrome and the treatment of these conditions by lifestyle modification.

- Arrange follow-up tests and review in four to six weeks.

Interpersonal skills:

This case tests the doctor's ability to explore the patient's understanding of a new diagnosis and to build on his existing ideas to develop a targeted and shared management plan.

Good communication with the patient:

- explores what the patient already knows and understands about his health.

- highlights issues the patient prioritises, such as 'lack of interest in cooking' and 'too much meat'. Therefore, the doctor provides focused information and advice, using motivational interviewing skills.

- negotiates which diagnostic tests are needed and justifies why some investigations (such as the X-ray) are not currently indicated.

- links the clinical presentation of gout with the abnormal blood tests.

- explains the global picture of increased cardiovascular risk to the patient in simple terms.

Poor communication with the patient:

- does not enquire sufficiently about his health understanding (gout, meat, alcohol).

- instructs the patient rather than seeking common ground (lectures the patient on alcohol units and calories without establishing what is realistic for him).

- uses inappropriate or technical language (in explaining the abnormal blood test results).

- appears patronising or inappropriately paternalistic (when discussing the management plan).

BACKGROUND KNOWLEDGE REQUIRED FOR THIS CASE

Epidemiology of gout

Doherty, M (2008) **New insights into the epidemiology of gout**. *Rheumatology*, **48**, supplement, pii2–ii8.

The usual initial presentation of gout is with rapidly developing acute inflammatory monoarthritis, typically affecting the first MTP joint. If left untreated it may progress with recurrent acute attacks and eventual development of chronic symptoms and joint damage. Several risk factors for gout can be modified to improve patient outcomes.

The dietary risk factors for gout are higher intakes of red meat, fructose and beer, all independently associated with increased risk, whereas higher intakes of coffee, low-fat dairy products and vitamin C are associated with lower risk. Many drugs influence serum uric acid levels through an effect on renal urate transport.

Comorbidities, including the metabolic syndrome and impaired renal function, are common in gout patients.

Metabolic syndrome

Khunti, K and Davies, M (2005) **Metabolic syndrome**, *BMJ*, **331**: 1153–1154.

What is metabolic syndrome?

Metabolic syndrome is characterised by hyper-insulinaemia, low glucose tolerance, dyslipidaemia, hypertension, and obesity, conditions that increase the risk of developing heart disease and diabetes.

What does it look like?

The clinical identification of metabolic syndrome is based on measures of:

- abdominal obesity,
- atherogenic dyslipidaemia,
- hypertension, and
- glucose intolerance.

Clinical criteria

People meeting three of the following criteria qualify as having the metabolic syndrome:

- raised blood pressure (>130/85mmHg),
- a low serum concentration of HDL cholesterol (<1.04mmol/L in men and <1.29 mmol/L in women),
- a high serum triglyceride concentration (>1.69mmol/L),

- a high fasting plasma glucose concentration (>6.1mmol/L), and
- abdominal obesity (waist circumference >102 cm in men and >88 cm in women). A new definition has central obesity as an essential criterion, with a range of cut-offs for waist circumference for people from different ethnic groups.

Lifestyle changes

Advice from the University of Southampton School of Medicine:
www.metabolicsyndrome.org.uk/Treatment/default.htm

- The risk of developing the metabolic syndrome increases with weight gain. Therefore, weight loss is one of the cornerstones of management. The general aim is to decrease calorie intake while increasing energy expenditure.

- Cycling or jogging 3 times a week over 20 to 26 weeks has been found to reduce cholesterol by 14% and triglycerides by 34%, while doubling HDL.

- There is some evidence that specific dietary changes can have benefits in addition to weight loss alone.
  - Eat more dietary fibre and consume less dietary fat.
  - Replace dietary saturated fats with equal amounts of unsaturated fats to lower LDL cholesterol and triglycerides.
  - Eat foods with a low glycaemic index – by slowing digestion and absorption, they have much less of a dyslipidaemic effect.

Relevant literature

For a good patient information sheet, see
http://www.ukgoutsociety.org/PDFs/goutsocietyhealthproblemsfinal2011.pdf

CASE 5 Hypertensive with gout

INFORMATION FOR THE DOCTOR

Name	Michael Abbot
Age	52
Social and family history	Married, two adult children
Past medical history	• Gout 8 weeks ago • Hypertension for five years; ankle swelling with amlodipine • Stomach upset and mood swings on statins – refuses statins • GORD 15 years ago
Current medication	• Ramipril 10mg daily • Hydrochlorothiazide 25mg daily • Naproxen 750mg stat followed by 250mg every 8 hours
Blood tests Plasma urate (2 years ago) CRP Plasma fasting glucose Fasting cholesterol Fasting HDL cholesterol Total cholesterol:HDL Fasting triglyceride* TSH Alkaline phosphatase Total bilirubin Albumin Creatinine level U&Es BMI BP	*Blood tests done last week* 632 (210–480) 8 (<8) 5.8mmol/L (3.65–5.5) 7.2mmol/L 0.8mmol/l (0.8–1.8) 9 2.9 (0.55–1.9) 1.89 (0.35–5.5) 156IU/L (95–280) 14µmol/L (3–17) 46g/L (35–50) 99µmol/L (70–150) within the normal range 29 146/86 (patient says home readings are consistently <140/90)

INFORMATION FOR THE PATIENT

You are Michael Abbot, a 52-year-old logistics manager, who has come to discuss the blood tests you had last week. The doctor you saw two months ago with a painful left foot suspected gout. She advised you to take anti-inflammatories and to return for a blood test 6–8 weeks after the attack settled. The doctor wanted to confirm her diagnosis of gout by doing the blood tests.

You had a very painful left foot with a swollen joint which was incredibly sore to touch. The skin was red and tender. For a week, you could hardly bear to put weight on it. The medication prescribed did help. You can now walk without difficulty, whereas when it first started, the pain had limited walking and any pressure put through the foot was agonising.

The doctor who advised getting a blood test to see if your uric acid was raised warned you not to get the test too soon after the first attack. You read about gout and your internet searching also advised getting a uric acid test 6 weeks after the attack. You expect the blood test to show a raised uric acid. You have read the advice about decreasing red meat and alcohol and want to know if this really works or whether you should just be put on tablets to prevent further attacks.

You present to the doctor expecting to discuss the blood tests and their implications. Your opening statement is *"I've come to discuss my blood tests"*.

Information to reveal if asked

General information about yourself:

- You work at a large logistics company. You take the train to and from work.
- When you were unwell with the painful foot, you could not walk to and from the train station and spent 5 days working from home. It was not the same as being in the office and you had to catch up with work on your return.
- You tend to socialise with colleagues; this usually involves some drinking after work.
- You have never smoked tobacco.

Further details about your condition:

- The foot pain two months ago was your first episode of gout. You do not have a family history of gout. Your dad died of a heart attack at the age of 68, but he smoked heavily. Your younger brother also has hypertension.
- If specifically asked about your lifestyle, you are a non-smoker. You drink no more than 3 pints of beer with colleagues 2–3 nights per week. You share a bottle of wine with your wife on most weekends. You tend to drink most nights,

either wine with a meal or beer with colleagues. You don't drink to get drunk and rarely drink more than a bottle of wine on your own or more than 6 pints of beer in one night.

- You and your wife like cooking and eating. You like red meat. You enjoy doing a roast dinner every weekend.

- You like vegetables but don't consider salads or vegetarian food a proper main course.

Your ideas:

- You think that your foot pain was gout. You suspect that you may have to change your diet and eat less meat, but how much meat should you be eating? Is oily fish OK?

- You don't think that you drink heavily.

- In the past, the doctor tried you on two different statins, but even on small doses you experienced a 'dodgy stomach' and vile mood swings. When you stopped the statin, the symptoms disappeared and when you restarted, they recurred. You discussed the risks and benefits of statins and decided that you didn't want to take them.

- You developed ankle swelling with a previous BP tablet. You have been reluctant to take more tablets or increase the dosage of current medication because of your experience of drug side-effects.

- You have read about medication to prevent attacks of gout, but you'd prefer not to take a daily tablet.

- If the doctor offers to swap one tablet for another, rather than prescribe more tablets, you are more amenable. You'd like to know about possible side-effects.

- You don't think you are motivated enough to lose weight. You and your wife enjoy cooking, good food and going out to nice restaurants.

Your concerns:

- You are worried about taking daily tablets in case you develop side-effects.

- If you have to change your diet, your wife will be affected. It will be impossible to go out with her, or cook her a nice meal, and then eat salad while she has a steak.

Your expectations:

- You expect to get information about the blood tests and have a discussion about treatments for gout.

Medical history

You consider yourself to be 'in good nick'. Your home blood pressure monitoring shows your BP to be well controlled despite it always being a bit high in surgery. You do not currently have any side-effects from your BP tablets.

Social history

You are happily married and your two adult children live away from home.

You enjoy your current social life.

Information to reveal if examined

If the doctor asks to do your blood pressure, hand him/her a card saying "BP consistently just slightly above 140/90".

SUGGESTED APPROACH TO THE CONSULTATION

Targeted history taking:

- What are Michael's symptoms now? What was his response to the anti-inflammatories? Did he experience any side-effects from the anti-inflammatories?

- Does he know why the blood tests were requested? What does he make of the raised uric acid? Does he have any ideas about how uric acid could be reduced? What would be the long-term effect of a raised uric acid?

- What are his concerns? Is he worried that his current social life, which revolves around food and alcohol, needs to be altered and the knock-on effect this will have on friends and family?

- What are his expectations: does he expect specific dietary and lifestyle advice; signposting to diets for patients with gout; medication?

- Is he prepared to revisit his risk factors for cardiovascular disease? He is not reaching target for cholesterol and BMI.

- Is he prepared to change his hypertension medication?

Targeted examination:

- This case does not require the candidate to perform a targeted physical examination.

Clinical management:

- Discuss the blood results and previous examination findings: he has a raised serum urate, cholesterol, triglycerides and BMI, all risk factors for CV disease.

- Discuss the risk of recurrent attacks of gout and the potential damage to several joints.

- Discuss what could be done about the raised uric acid: reduction in alcohol consumption (especially beer and spirits); reduction in meat, seafood and food containing fructose (corn syrup); losing weight; exercising more; changing his BP tablets from hydrochlorothiazide to losartan; optimising his BP and cholesterol treatments. Of these options, which one would he like to try first? Discuss that uric acid-reducing medication such as allopurinol is usually offered to patients who suffer two or more attacks of acute gout in a year.

- Address the patient's ideas: that it is too difficult to make lifestyle changes. Negotiate goals for Michael to work towards and ask him what help he may need in reaching these goals. Consider referral to the practice nurse for healthy eating and lifestyle advice.

- Address the patient's concerns about prophylactic daily medication and making drastic lifestyle changes. If he stops hydrochlorothiazide, which can increase uric acid by 20%, and if he starts losartan, which can decrease uric acid by up to 20%, he may reduce his risk gout, improve his BP control and reduce the number of pills he takes.

- Address the patient's expectations about pill side-effects.

- Confirm his understanding of gout, its immediate treatment with anti-inflammatories (does he have a standby supply?), its link with cardiovascular disease and the treatment of these conditions by lifestyle modification.

- Arrange follow-up in four weeks to check BP and revisit cardiovascular risk factors.

Interpersonal skills:

This case tests the doctor's ability to negotiate with a patient to develop a shared management plan. It also tests the doctor's ability to maintain an adult–adult relationship with a patient who is so reluctant to make lifestyle changes that his behaviour borders on teenage stroppiness.

Good communication with the patient:

- explores what the patient already knows and helps the patient to assimilate the new information to make his own decisions. The doctor could ask *"If you did nothing about your drinking, diet and exercise, what is the worst that could happen? If you made all the lifestyle changes, what is the best that could happen? What are the most realistic changes that you could make? If you had a friend in this situation, what would you advise him to do?"*

- Once the patient has committed to making some changes, the doctor gives focused information, support and follow-up.

- Good prescribing behaviour involves discussing how to discontinue current BP tablets and to start the new medication.

Poor communication with the patient:

- does not enquire sufficiently about his health understanding and sees his reluctance to make changes as being a stroppy or difficult patient. The poor communicator adopts a parent–child approach.

- instructs the patient. Instead of motivating the patient to change, the poor communicator lectures the patient on alcohol units and purine-rich food. Hence, the doctor appears patronising or inappropriately paternalistic.

- uses inappropriate or technical language (in explaining the test results and treatment options, including medication).

BACKGROUND KNOWLEDGE REQUIRED FOR THIS CASE

Suresh, E (2005) **Diagnosis and management of gout**. *Postgrad. Med. J.* **81**: s572–579. doi:10.1136/pgmj.2004.030692

There are three prerequisites for development of gout:

- Development of hyperuricaemia leading to urate saturation;
- Formation of monosodium urate crystals;
- Interactions between monosodium urate crystals and leucocytes.

Secondary causes of hyperuricaemia include:

- chronic renal failure
- ingestion of drugs that compete with urate for renal excretion including loop or thiazide diuretics, low-dose aspirin, or cyclosporin.
- Patients sometimes know when an acute episode is imminent, describing itching (possibly caused by prodromal mast cell degranulation and release of histamine).
- Acute episodes often begin at night – hence the suggestion "suspect gout when acute arthritis begins between 2 and 7am."
- The episode builds to a peak over several hours with intense pain and increased sensitivity of overlying skin such that even pressure of bed covers cannot be tolerated.
- The reason for extreme pain in acute gout is unknown.
- Gout affects the first MTP joint in >70% of cases but other joints such as tarsal joints, ankles, knees, and wrists can also be affected. Central joints such as hips, shoulders, and spine are seldom affected, possibly because higher temperatures in these joints are not conducive to crystallisation.
- It is unclear why only one or two joints are affected at a time, but occasionally episodes can be polyarticular, especially later in the course of the disease.
- Fever is common and more likely with polyarticular episodes (in about 50%).
- Gout can also cause bursitis and tenosynovitis.
- Resolution is usual within a week, even without treatment.

Diet, drinking, and diuretics (correctable risk factors)

- An increased risk of gout was found with increased meat consumption (particularly beef, pork, lamb and seafood) but not with consumption of purine-rich vegetables.
- A rigid purine-free diet is, however, unpalatable, impractical, and can rarely be sustained.

- Serum urate concentrations and frequency of episodes can be reduced by weight reduction through calorie restriction, decreased intake of carbohydrates, and increased proportional intake of protein and unsaturated fat. Such a diet would also decrease plasma glucose, insulin, and triglyceride concentrations and improve insulin sensitivity, thereby reducing cardiovascular morbidity and mortality.
- Crash dieting and fasting should be avoided as they can precipitate acute episodes.
- Excess consumption of alcohol should be discouraged, as increasing alcohol intake is associated with an increasing risk of gout. Beer confers a larger risk than spirits, but moderate wine drinking does not seem to increase the risk of gout.
- Consider alternatives to diuretic therapy.

CASE 6 Overactive bladder

INFORMATION FOR THE DOCTOR

Name	Maya Tunstill
Age	49
Past medical history	• GORD – on lansoprazole 15mg once daily (3 months ago) • Insertion copper IUD (5 years ago) • Carpal tunnel right (8 years ago)
Test results U&Es, fasting glucose (3 months ago) Cervical smear BMI BP	 normal normal 24 132/84

INFORMATION FOR THE PATIENT

You are 49-year-old Maya Tunstill. You recently read a magazine article about Botox injections for overactive bladders and think that you need this treatment. For the last seven years, you have had problems with your wee. Initially you thought you were getting bladder infections, but the antibiotics did not help and the wee samples never grew any bugs. You thought that you go so often (every two hours) because you drank coffee, but cutting out caffeine made no difference. When your bladder is full, you have a strong desire to go and cannot really delay for longer than ten minutes. You have to cross your legs when you insert the key into your front door lock and rush to the toilet on entering the house. Sometimes you don't make it to the toilet on time and your knickers are damp. You find that you wake once at night to pass urine, but on returning to bed, fall off to sleep quite quickly. These were all the symptoms described in the magazine. The woman writing the article advised that Botox has completely changed the lives of women affected by urinary symptoms like yours. You had not heard of Botox for urine symptoms before but if it is as good as the article described, then you'd like to know more.

You present to the doctor to discuss Botox for your urine symptoms. Your opening statement is *"I've come to ask for your advice about Botox for my bladder doctor"*.

Information to reveal if asked

General information about yourself:

- You are a part-time receptionist at a local car dealership.

- You read about the Botox in an article about a woman who, after she had Botox, bought a new car, and now enjoys her long road trips.

- You are very happy with your copper coil. Its insertion made no difference to your urinary symptoms.

- Your family is complete. You have two children aged 17 and 22.

Further details about your condition:

- When your bladder is full, you feel uncomfortable and find yourself wiggling about in your chair, but you do not have any pain on passing urine.

- You have not noticed passing blood in your urine.

- You have not had kidney stones.

- You had normal deliveries and you have not had any abdominal or pelvic surgery.

- Your bowels are absolutely fine.

- You do not have a significant family history other than your mum developed hypertension at the age of 72.

Your ideas:

- You think that your symptoms are not due to caffeine or bladder infections as previous doctors had assumed. It is something that happens to the bladder as women get older, especially if they have had children.

Your concerns:

- You expect to get information about Botox for bladder symptoms but you are worried that the article sounded too good to be true, so you'd like your GP to give you an independent opinion.

- You are worried that if the bladder gets older and the symptoms get worse, then the Botox won't be able to help any more. Should you treat it before it gets worse or results in permanent damage?

Your expectations:

- You think it may be a common problem for women as they get older but if Botox could make the bladder behave as if it were young again, you'd consider it, but you'd like to know how the Botox is inserted into the bladder and what the risks are.

Medical history

You are in good general health, and are not on long-term medication. You are not particularly worried about having an operation.

Social history

You have two children and your family is complete. Your husband is not disturbed by your night-time trips to the bathroom. Your family moan about the need to stop often at motorway service stations for loo breaks but this problem has not restricted you in any way.

You enjoy spicy food and diet drinks.

Information to reveal if examined

Abdominal examination – no masses palpable; soft and non-tender.

SUGGESTED APPROACH TO THE CONSULTATION

Targeted history taking:

- What are her bladder symptoms? Ascertain if Mrs Tunstill has urgency, frequency, nocturia and/or incontinence.

- Are there any symptoms of stress incontinence?

- Are there any specific reasons why she is more likely to have detrusor overactivity, such as neurological problems (Parkinson's, stroke, dementia, multiple sclerosis, diabetic neuropathy)?

- What are her ideas about what is happening to her bladder to produce her current symptoms?

- What are her concerns? Is she worried that these symptoms may herald the onset of other illness, such as menopausal symptoms (oestrogen deficiency-induced atropy) or bladder cancer? Is she concerned that if she did nothing about her present symptoms, the problem would get worse or result in irreparable damage to the bladder?

- What are her expectations? Clearly she wants information about Botox (availability; her suitability for treatment, effectiveness; side-effects; referral) but is she certain about her diagnosis and has she considered alternative treatments for the condition?

- Has she heard of bladder retraining or anti-cholinergic medication?

- Does she have any general health problems, or is she on any medication, that would make conservative management difficult?

- What does she already know about lifestyle changes (caffeine reduction), bladder retraining (scheduled voiding), medication (anti-cholinergic drugs) and Botox?

Targeted examination:

- Based on her notes, she is not overweight and has normal renal function (checked 3 months ago).

- Ask to perform a brief, targeted abdominal examination.

Clinical management:

- Address the patient's ideas: she believes that she has a common age-related bladder problem. Use the patient's ideas to develop and explain the pathology of overactive bladder syndrome, the most likely diagnosis. But, the suspicion of overactive bladder syndrome needs to be confirmed first, so it is important to gather more information to make the correct diagnosis before discussing therapy.

- You may advise Mrs Tunstill to complete a bladder diary for a minimum of three days and to do a urinary dipstix.

- Mrs Tunstill has a specific concern that if she does nothing about this problem, the bladder will get damaged and symptoms will worsen. If the problem is an overactive bladder syndrome, then doing nothing is an option. She does not need treatment if her symptoms do not significantly interfere with her quality of life. She will also need to balance the risk of any treatment for overactive bladder syndrome with its potential benefits. If her bladder diary indicates overactive bladder syndrome, then options are do nothing; make lifestyle changes; do bladder retraining; take anti-cholinergic medication; or have Botox. If her quality of life at present is good, does she want to take the risks associated with medication (dry mouth, constipation) or Botox (possible need for intermittent self-catheterisation, need for more than one injection, increased risk of UTIs)?

- Address Mrs Tunstill's expectations: she expects for her bladder condition to be taken seriously – she hinted at this by suggesting an invasive treatment such as Botox as a treatment possibility. Negotiate expectations by explaining the need for correct diagnosis first. Then the pros and cons of the treatment options can be discussed so she can make an informed decision about how she would like to tackle the issue.

Interpersonal skills:

This case tests the doctor's ability to develop a shared management plan. The patient has presented with a solution to a self-diagnosed problem. The trick is for the doctor to make his or her own diagnosis without offending the patient. One approach could be *"Mrs Tunstill, I know you came to talk about Botox for bladder problems, but could I just check that we are talking about the same bladder condition? Just to clarify things for me, I need to ask you a few questions about your symptoms"*. By doing this, the doctor has subtly altered the agenda from a discussion on Botox to a discussion about the diagnosis.

If this negotiation over agenda takes place early and is done smoothly, Mrs Tunstill may feel that the doctor is working with her to seek the best treatment for her. The discussion about bladder diaries is then more likely to be met with approval rather than seen as an attempt to avoid the Botox discussion. The discussion could continue along the lines of *"If the bladder diaries point to a diagnosis of overactive bladder syndrome, then yes, Botox may be an option but there are also some very good tablets we can discuss. Unlike Botox, tablets are much easier to start and much easier to stop if there are problems. Also, the tablets have been studied for a lot longer, so we have a lot more information about long-term effectiveness and safety, which I know are important considerations for you"*. Mrs Tunstill is more likely to see such a discussion as having her interests at heart.

BACKGROUND KNOWLEDGE REQUIRED FOR THIS CASE

Relevant literature

http://pathways.nice.org.uk/pathways/urinary-incontinence-in-women
(3 Sept 2014)

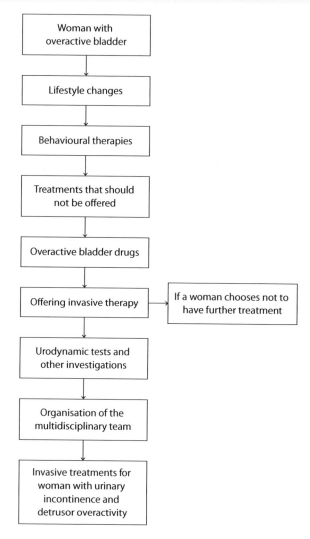

CASE 7 Sick note

INFORMATION FOR THE DOCTOR

Name	Glenda Hughes
Age	46
Past medical history	Hypertension for the last three years

The medical record for her **last consultation** three months ago when she was seen by the practice nurse for a BP check, reads:

"Never smoked tobacco. 4 units alcohol per week. No side-effects with medication. No new symptoms. Blood withdrawal from L antecubital fossa with patient's consent. Will be informed of test results in writing. Will make appointment to see GP in six months for BP check and repeat prescription."

Test results	
U&Es	normal
Fasting glucose	normal
BMI	24.6
BP	132/76
Cervical smear	normal

INFORMATION FOR THE PATIENT

You are 46-year-old Glenda Hughes. You rarely come to the Surgery except for your blood pressure checks. You feel that the surgery has looked after you well and helped you to understand and control your BP problems. You find the surgery staff helpful.

You consult today because you were unable to work your Friday late-night shift – you had a cold. However, on your return to work (you are a part-time carer), the Care Agency boss demanded a sick note. She seemed to imply that Friday night was a 'convenient' time to get ill. The Care Agency is short-staffed and when you called in ill, the Agency had difficulty finding someone else at short notice. You are very apologetic for consulting but you don't know what to do. Your line manager was quite aggressive and you are somewhat upset that you were not believed, but you also do not want to make things worse at work by not providing a sick note.

You didn't consult with the doctors on Friday because you knew the cold would resolve spontaneously. You spent most of the weekend in bed and felt and looked much better on Monday when you returned to work. By the time of today's consultation, the cold has resolved spontaneously and you look and sound normal.

You present for a sick note. You do not like or trust your line manager; she has favourites and she picks on some people. You would prefer not to challenge or confront her for fear of her picking on you in future.

Your opening statement is *"I'm so sorry to trouble you doctor, but my boss insists that I need a sick note for last Friday"*.

Information to reveal if asked

- You are married with two teenage girls.

- You do thirty hours per week as a Carer, usually the evening shifts when your girls are back from school. You have worked for the Care Agency for four years and like the work. A new manager was put in place six months ago and she has introduced efficiency measures. The climate at work has changed. People are less happy and are being questioned more about what they do, how they do it and if things can be done with fewer resources. Some people have left. You like your clients and you would like to continue working. You just want to keep your head down and carry on quietly.

Further details about your condition:

- You had a cold: headache, sore throat, nasal congestion and sniffles, feeling generally weak with muscle ache. You started to feel unwell on Wednesday during work; it worsened on Thursday, your day off and was starting to improve on Friday but you felt that if you went to work, you'd pass your illness to other people and you may relapse from exerting yourself too soon.

- You are usually fit and healthy. You can't remember the last time you had time off work.

Your ideas:

- You think your line manager is being unreasonable but she isn't a particularly nice person, so you are not surprised by her request.

- You are surprised if the doctor tells you that you cannot get a sick note and want an explanation for this. You don't trouble the surgery much and feel that they should understand your dilemma and help you out. You didn't need to be seen when ill; you knew you had a cold and you knew you needed to rest, have fluids and take paracetamol for fever. You believe that the surgery could give you a back-dated sick note. Writing the note will take a few minutes, so although you don't like wasting the doctor's time, you don't see yourself as taking up much time. If the doctor discusses writing a letter for your employer you are OK with that. If the doctor talks to you about there being a fee for the letter, you are surprised and want to know what the fee is for and how much it will cost.

Your concerns:

- You are concerned about what is written on the note. You prefer the wording to be *"Viral upper respiratory tract infection"* or *"I certify that Mrs Glenda Hughes was unable to attend work because she had a cold"*.

- If the doctor writes something like *"Mrs Glenda Hughes tells me she was unable to attend work because she had a cold"* you ask the doctor to reword the letter.

Your expectations:

- You want to leave with the sick note and cannot come back later to collect it.

- If asked to pay, you think anything more than £10 is really quite expensive, seeing as it will only take the doctor a few minutes to write it. You want an explanation about why a retrospective note cannot be issued.

Medical history

Apart from well-controlled hypertension, you are in good general health.

Social history

You are married with two children.

You want to keep this job. When you stayed at home when the girls were little, you found you became a bit isolated and low. This job, even though it has its challenges, forces you to leave the house and interact with people. Last year, you used some of your own savings to go on holiday to Turkey with your sister and mother.

Information to reveal if examined

You look well. Your BP is 139/75 (if taken).

SUGGESTED APPROACH TO THE CONSULTATION

Targeted history taking:

- Why does Mrs Hughes require a sick note: what illness, what were her symptoms; what was the duration of illness; when did she recover? Is she well now?

- The doctor also obtains sufficient information to assess if her health-seeking behaviour was appropriate: how did you treat yourself?

- Why does her boss want a sick note?

- What are the circumstances like at work?

- What does she think of being made to attend for a note?

- What does she know about regulations regarding certification for minor illness?

Targeted examination:

- Examination is not required in this case.

Clinical management:

- Address the patient's ideas – she believes that it is better to ask for a retrospective sick note for minor illness than it is to confront her line manager. She may not realise that by law only self-certification is required for the first seven days of illness.

- If an employee requires a 'fit note' for an illness of less than seven days' duration, then a doctor's statement in a letter may be provided. In 2014, the BMA-recommended fee for 'a straightforward certificate of fact' is £17.50, to be met either by the patient or the employer. By asking for a sick note fee to cover the administrative costs of providing the note, the message GPs are sending to employers and employees is that it is inappropriate to ask GPs to provide sick notes to cover minor illness. Employers (and Mrs Hughes' manager) cannot expect GPs to police sickness absence. The NHS has a finite number of resources and stretching these resources to provide a cheap occupational health service to private companies reduces the time available for seeing and treating ill patients. Providing 'free' doctor's letters could encourage patients to attend for minor illness, thereby promoting inappropriate health-seeking behaviour. If letters are provided free of charge to patients with minor illness, the practice appointments could be inundated with patients requesting letters, which is an inappropriate use of resources.

- Address the patient's concerns about what is written on the fit note. In its guidance to GPs on how to complete the fit note, GPs are advised to *"Describe the condition(s) that affect your patient's fitness for work. Give as accurate a diagnosis as possible, unless you think a precise diagnosis will damage your patient's wellbeing or position with their employer."* Department of Work and Pensions,

Getting the most out of your fit note: GP Guidance (Jan 2014). www.gov.uk/
government/uploads/system/uploads/attachment_data/file/298821/fitnote-
gps-guidance-jan-14.pdf

- Fulfil her expectations for a note: with a good explanation or with a fit note or
  with a private letter. If you complete the fit note make sure to fill in the dates
  correctly. Fill in the date on which the case was first assessed (today's date) and
  today's date in the 'date of the statement' section. In the section two lines above
  the doctor's signature ("This will be the case from … to …"), put in the start and
  end dates of the illness. If you provide a GP letter, ensure that it complies with
  the principles governing fit notes.

Interpersonal skills:

Good communication and negotiation with the patient involves making the care of
your patient your first concern.

- Make sure that your patient is well. Take the time to understand her situation.
  Empathise with her difficulties.

- But it is also important to encourage appropriate health-seeking behaviour. So
  praise Mrs Hughes for acting appropriately when she developed a self-limiting
  illness. Unlike her manager, she behaved correctly.

Ethical and professional conduct encompasses protecting and promoting the
health of patients and the public.

- **Use resources appropriately**: GPs can only protect and promote health if they
  have sufficient resources, such as appointment times. Where they have limited
  resources, then they need to take steps to ensure that these are distributed first
  to those patients with the greatest need. Therefore, to protect the health of their
  patients, they need to distribute their appointments appropriately. GPs would be
  failing in this duty if they permitted their surgeries to be cluttered with sick note
  requests for minor illnesses.

- **Treat patients as individuals and respect their dignity**: Treat patients politely
  and considerately – it is appropriate for GPs to take steps to discourage sick
  note requests. It is also appropriate to listen to Mrs Hughes and to explain the
  appropriate use of sick notes. Getting angry, sarcastic, rude or offensive would
  be impolite and inconsiderate.

Respect patients' right to confidentiality – be careful and truthful in what you write
on a fit note or private letter.

Work in partnership with patients

- Listen to patients and respond to their concerns and preferences: it would
  be incorrect to simply brush aside Mrs Hughes' request with *"I don't write sick
  notes for sickness absence lasting less than a week. That is the law. Goodbye."* It is

important to discharge your responsibilities in listening and responding to her concerns and preferences. But that response could be a good explanation and a show of empathy rather than acceding to her request. You need to maintain your doctor–patient relationship, but you also need to educate Mrs Hughes about your duties as a doctor and justify to her from a professional and legal standpoint the reasons for your actions.

- Give patients the information they want or need in a way they can understand. You need to word your explanation to suit Mrs Hughes' level of understanding. If she fails to understand, then you have failed in your duty to communicate effectively. Understanding information is different to accepting or believing that information. Your responsibility is getting her to understand the information, so use everyday language if you are going to explain ethical concepts.

Be honest and open and act with integrity

- Never discriminate unfairly against patients or colleagues – it would be unfair of you to refuse to issue a sick note to Mrs Hughes but to issue one to another patient with whom you are friends or from whom you fear a complaint. The sick note policy should apply equally to all patients. You could direct Mrs Hughes to the Practice Policy.

- Never abuse your patients' trust in you or the public's trust in the profession. For example, back-dating a sick note, or making up a reason for the patient's illness, is an abuse of the public's trust in the profession.

BACKGROUND KNOWLEDGE REQUIRED FOR THIS CASE

Department of Work and Pensions, *Getting the most out of your fit note: GP Guidance* (Jan 2014).

Filling in the fit note

You can issue a fit note on the day that you assess your patient; or on any day afterwards.

The fit note should be completed as follows:

1. Write the date on which you assessed your patient. This can be via a face-to-face or telephone consultation; or consideration of a written report from another doctor or healthcare professional (for example, nurses, occupational therapists, physiotherapists).

2. Describe the condition(s) that affect your patient's fitness for work. Give as accurate a diagnosis as possible, unless you think a precise diagnosis will damage your patient's wellbeing or position with their employer.

3. Tick 'not fit for work' OR 'may be fit for work taking account of the following advice'.

4. The comments box must be completed when you tick 'may be fit for work'. Completion is optional if you have ticked 'not fit for work'.

5. Indicate the period that your advice applies for. This may be the date that you expect your patient to have recovered by, or your judgement about an appropriate time to review their fitness for work even if they are unlikely to have fully recovered.

6. Sign the fit note using ink.

7. Complete the date of statement. This is the date that you issue the fit note.

Your patient can go back to work at any point they feel able to, even if this is before their fit note expires. They do not need to come back to see you in order to do so, or get a new fit note. This is the case even if you have indicated that you need to assess them again.

How your patient will use their fit note

1. If your patient is employed and you have indicated that that they are not fit for work, they can use the fit note to claim sick pay. Your patient should keep their original fit note and their employer may take a copy for their records.

2. If your patient is employed and you have indicated that they may be fit for work, they should discuss your advice with their employer to see if there are changes which could support them to return to work (for example changing their duties, adjusting work premises or providing special equipment). You do not need to suggest any of these changes – your advice is purely on the impact of your patient's health condition and it is up to your patient and their employer to discuss ways to accommodate it. If their employer cannot make any changes to accommodate your advice, the fit note is treated as if it stated that your patient was not fit for work. Your patient should not return to you for a new fit note stating this because they do not need one.

3. If your patient is out of work, they can use a fit note to support a claim for health-related benefits or to show that they have been unable to fulfil certain benefit requirements. They can also use it in any discussions with prospective employers about supporting a health condition.

CASE 8 Unwell insulin-dependent diabetic

INFORMATION FOR THE DOCTOR

This is a telephone consultation.

Name	Michael Ede
Age	29
Past medical history	• Type 1 diabetes 2 years ago • Patello-femoral knee joint pain syndrome 4 years ago

The medical record of his **last consultation** last month, when he was seen by the practice nurse, reads:

"Patient was diagnosed with type 1 diabetes two years ago. His diabetic control is good and his recent IFCC A1C was 56.

Has had flu vaccination previously with no problems. Comes for flu vaccination today. Offered pneumococcal vaccination – accepted.

Patient is able to self-monitor his blood glucose and is well-educated and motivated in diabetes self-care. Will telephone for advice if develops side-effects to vaccination."

Current medication	• Levemir pen fill injections 100units/ml • Novorapid pen fill cartridges 100units/ml • Novo pens 3 and 4: 1–60units • Glucose oral gel 40% • Glucagen Hypokit injection 1mg • Test strips • Ketone strips

INFORMATION FOR THE PATIENT

You are Michael Ede, a 29-year-old engineer. You were diagnosed with Type 1 diabetes after a sudden short illness 2 years ago. Since the diagnosis you have taken a very proactive approach to optimising your blood sugar management. Over the past year your insulin control has improved – you had 3 episodes of hypoglycaemia in the first year but you have not had any episodes of hypoglycaemia in the last year. You check your BG 8 to 10 times per day.

You are calling the GP today because you became suddenly unwell during the night and seek advice on adjusting your insulin. Since 1 am you felt unwell: it started with feeling hot, then cold, shivering and sweating. Then the diarrhoea and vomiting started – fluid, no blood, on the hour. You last vomited two hours ago, after which you checked your BG. It was 9. You have been taking sips of water, but feel unable to eat.

Your opening statement is *"I've got pretty bad D&V doctor, but Dioralyte and squashes have too much sugar. What should I drink?"*

Information to reveal if asked

General information about yourself:

- You were part of the University research trial and learnt on a two-week residential course a huge amount on how to match your carbohydrate requirements with exercise demands.

- You are physically very active. Since the course, you exercise for one hour per day, 5 days per week and you have not had any episodes of disabling hypoglycaemia. You also have normal awareness of hypoglycaemic symptoms. When you feel your blood glucose dropping (a vague sensation) you test yourself. If BG is <4, you are able to treat yourself with dextrose tablets and you recover quickly.

- Your work has made adjustments to your engineering job. You don't work at heights and you don't work alone on shifts. You tend to deal with work that is brought into the workshop; you do not drive to off-site calls. However, the company Occupational Medicine doctor advised you that your job will be reviewed if you start to have diabetes that is brittle and difficult to control. In particular, the company is worried about hypoglycaemia and the risk it poses to your ability to handle certain machinery or sign off safety-critical work.

Further details about your condition:

- You think you ate 'something bad' and developed food poisoning or an infectious illness.

- You feel 'dehydrated' – you have been to the toilet every hour and passed 'water'. You have been vomiting a lot but in the last two hours, you felt less nauseated.
- You have a few lower abdominal cramps when you pass stool but you do not have severe abdominal pain or urinary symptoms.
- You have not vomited blood or passed blood rectally.

Your ideas:

- You should rehydrate with something but you are not sure what fluid would be best.
- Should you take Dioralyte or squash and insulin?
- If you are not eating, should you cut your insulin?

Your concerns:

- You do not want to have hypoglycaemia because it has repercussions for work. You do not want to spoil your HbA1c reading next month.

Your expectations:

- You cannot get hold of your diabetic nurse at the University Hospital; you left a message for her to call back. In the interim, you expect the GP to give specific advice on how to rehydrate, what to eat and how much insulin to take. You do not recall being issued a copy of 'sick day rules'.

Medical history

2 years ago   Type 1 diabetes – sudden onset. You were told yours was an unusual presentation at your age.

4 years ago   Patello-femoral knee joint pain syndrome – exercise overuse from a three-week charity cycling event.

Social history

You got married a month ago. Your wife, who had the same sweet and sour chicken as you, is perfectly well.

Information to reveal if examined

Your last blood glucose was 9 and ketones trace (2 hours ago).

SUGGESTED APPROACH TO THE CONSULTATION

Targeted history taking:

- When did Michael last eat or drink? Is he able to keep down fluids? When did he last pass urine?
- Does he have any abdominal pain or urinary symptoms to suggest this is a more severe or different infection?
- Is he feeling so unwell or drowsy that he is unable to make good decisions?
- Is he able to monitor his blood glucose and ketones regularly?
- Is he alone? If he becomes more unwell, is there someone with him to look after him or call for help if he deteriorates?

Targeted examination:

- Not needed.

Clinical management:

- Manage the D&V: fluids, paracetamol if temperature or abdominal cramp, food as tolerated; anti-emetics if needed (buccal, oral tablets or injectables).
- Fluid: the type of fluid used as fluid replacement can be milky drinks or fruit juice, but if the patient is not eating solids, soups or cereals are good alternatives. Aim for 100ml of fluid every hour or approximately three litres in 24 hours.
- Food: try fish, meat, chicken or toast.
- Insulin and monitoring (blood glucose and ketones): as a rule of thumb, diabetics are more likely to have high blood glucose readings (hyperglycaemia) during an intercurrent illness so do not omit the insulin. Sometimes higher than normal doses of insulin are needed (see algorithm below). Test BG and blood ketones every 4 hours.
- Since Michael's last BG was 9 and blood ketones showed a trace only, he should take his usual dose of long-acting (bolus) insulin. He calculates his short-acting insulin dose in the usual way, based on the amount of carbohydrate he obtains from his intake of fluids (juice/soup) and food (fish, meat, chicken).
- He may require admission if:
  - the diarrhoea and vomiting are persistent.
  - blood glucose persistently >20mmol/L despite best therapy.
  - ketosis (+ and over) persists despite increasing the insulin dose or if the patient develops clinical signs of ketosis (e.g. Kussmaul's respiration, severe dehydration, abdominal pain).
  - the patient is unable to manage the sick day rules – poor understanding or too unwell to make sensible decisions.
  - it is unsafe to leave the patient alone, without social support where he may be at risk of slipping into unconsciousness.

Interpersonal skills:

This case tests the doctor's ability to assess and manage an 'emergency' presentation. The patient, though currently well, could become unwell quite quickly. The doctor needs to assess the situation systematically and make a diagnosis on probability. Even if the doctor does not have an emergency protocol to hand, he or she is able to give sensible advice (from first principles) on fluid, calories and insulin. The doctor is able to spell out for the patient the symptoms and signs that signal deterioration, so he is empowered to seek emergency care or admission; the doctor safety-nets appropriately.

Summary of information:

The patient monitors:

- Fluid intake
- Carbohydrate intake
- 4 hourly blood glucose
- 4 hourly blood ketones

List treatment:

- Fluid replacement
- Adequate carbohydrate and calorie intake
- Insulin usual or increased dose as determined by 4 hourly BG and blood ketones

BACKGROUND KNOWLEDGE REQUIRED FOR THIS CASE

NICE (CG15, July 2004) *Type 1 diabetes: guidance and guidelines*
www.nice.org.uk/guidance/cg15.CG

http://www.diabetes-support.org.uk/info/?page_id=141

Dafne uses two categories of illness: **minor**, where blood glucose levels are not too elevated and ketones don't appear as more than a trace, and **severe**, where BG levels are over 13 or ketones are present.

Minor:

If BG is less than 8mmol/L and ketones are negative:

- Maintain usual ratios of bolus insulin.
- Maintain usual basal doses.
- Monitor 4–6 hourly. (If you are not eating, you may only need the basal insulin.)

If BG is more than 8mmol/L and ketones are negative or trace:

- Maintain usual ratios of bolus insulin.
- Add corrective doses of bolus.
- Increase basal doses by 1–2 units (20%)
- Monitor 4–6 hourly. (If you are not eating, you may still need corrective bolus insulin.)

If BG is more than 13mmol/L and ketones are more than trace follow the "severe illness" rules.

Severe:

If BG is 10–13mmol/L and ketones are 'small' or 'moderate':

- Calculate the total insulin (basal and bolus) in the previous 24 hours, calculate 10% of that.
- Bolus: take equivalent of 10% of that daily total every 2 hours.
- Plus normal bolus ratio for anything you eat.
- Maintain usual basal doses. Monitor BG and ketones 2 hourly.
- Have 100ml of sugar-free liquids per hour.

When BG drops below 10mmol/L AND ketones are negative or trace:

- Eat/drink 10–20g carb.
- Use normal bolus ratios. Use normal basal dose.
- Monitor BG and ketones 2–4 hourly.

If BG is over 13mmol/L and ketones are 'moderate' or 'large':

- Calculate the total insulin (basal and bolus) in the previous 24 hours, calculate 20% of that.
- Bolus: take equivalent of 20% of that daily total every 2 hours, plus normal bolus ratio for anything you eat.
- Maintain usual basal doses.
- Monitor BG and ketones 2 hourly.
- Have 100ml of sugar-free liquids per hour.

When BG drops below 10mmol/L AND ketones are negative or trace:

- Eat/drink 10–20g carb.
- Use normal bolus ratios.
- Use normal basal dose.
- Monitor BG and ketones 2–4 hourly.

CASE 9 Termination of pregnancy

INFORMATION FOR THE DOCTOR

Name	Tiki Pham
Age	23
Past medical history	Not known – old GP notes have not yet arrived
Last consultation	New patient

INFORMATION FOR THE PATIENT

You are 23-year-old Tiki Pham. You did two home pregnancy tests, one last week when your period was a few days late and one yesterday. Both were positive. You suspect that you missed taking a few Microgynon pills at the time of your recent house move, when the Army posted your husband locally from Chepstow. Things at home have been hectic.

Your husband is a 21-year-old soldier and he has left, at short notice, on an overseas deployment two weeks ago. He is due back in two months. You telephoned your husband with news of the positive pregnancy tests. You both agree that you would currently find looking after another baby emotionally and financially difficult. Your husband got into debt with internet gambling, for which he sought help from the Army social services. Both of you have been advised on a financial plan.

You present requesting a termination of pregnancy. Your mind is made up. You want a referral to the TOP services.

Your opening statement is *"I've come to get a referral to the local Termination Clinic please"*.

Information to reveal if asked

General information about yourself:

- You are a 23-year-old mother of two boys aged 3 and 1. You do not think that giving the baby up for adoption is a consideration and you are adamant that you want a TOP. Also, given your current financial difficulties, you are worried about taking time off work from your new part-time job at the local supermarket.

- You have a car and can drive but travelling to an out-sourced centre would be difficult because of child care arrangements. Your family live in Fiji. You have not yet made friends locally. You do not want to tell anybody about your decision to have a TOP.

Further details about your condition that you reveal if directly asked:

- Both home pregnancy tests, which you trust, were positive. Based on the date of your last menstrual period, you calculate that you are five weeks pregnant. Your periods are usually very regular.

Your ideas:

- You think that the missed Pills (Microgynon) resulted in contraception failure.

- You want the TOP referral and do not want to be spoken to about other options. You do not have religious objections to TOP. You don't think that having a TOP results in any psychological or physical issues.

- However, you are worried about the post-treatment recovery times. You think you will need an operation under general anaesthetic (GA) at the local hospital, hopefully as a day case. You suspect you may need up to two weeks to recover.

- You are not aware of medical terminations.

Your concerns:

- You started working part-time in Waitrose last week and you are still in the probation period. If you are admitted to hospital, you don't know how you will tell your manager and how you will pay for child care. Your children are in nursery, using the nursery voucher scheme, while you work your Wednesday morning shift.

- In particular, you are concerned about after the procedure: will you be able to look after your sons and how much time off work will you need?

Your expectations:

- You want this doctor to understand that you have already made your decision and to provide the referral to the local TOP clinic. You want to know about the procedure, what symptoms you are likely to get after the procedure so you can make decisions about childcare and work. You haven't given any thought to what contraception you may need; your husband is away for several months and you have ample time to consider your contraception options.

Medical history

You are in good general health. Your two pregnancies were uneventful. Except for Microgynon, you are not on medication. You do not smoke.

Social history

Your family is complete. You'd like your husband to have a vasectomy but your last doctor told him he is too young and he can only have it done after the age of 30 years, which you think is ridiculous.

You are new to the Army camp and haven't made friends as yet.

Information to reveal if examined

You are not hypertensive or overweight. *Please have a card with your BP and weight.*

SUGGESTED APPROACH TO THE CONSULTATION

Targeted history taking:

- How does she know she is pregnant?
- Has she experienced failure of her regular contraception?
- When was her last menstrual period (LMP)? Are her periods usually regular?
- What are home circumstances like at the moment?
- On what grounds does she want a termination?
- Has she considered the options?
- How does her husband feel about her TOP request?
- Would having a termination impact on her home and work situation?
- Has she had a TOP before?
- What are her expectations of this consultation: a confirmation of her suspicions that she may be pregnant, a referral to the TOP service, advice on her options, or contraception advice for the future?
- Does she have any general health problems, or is she on any medication, that would make surgical or medical TOP unsafe?
- What does she already know about TOPs?
- If there are any logistical difficulties in arranging a TOP with the local hospital, could she travel further to an out-sourced TOP service?

Targeted examination:

- Based on her LMP, calculate the date of her pregnancy.
- Once you establish from your history that she definitely wants a referral for a TOP, you may want to provide a BP reading and BMI in your referral reading.

Clinical management:

- Address the patient's ideas: she believes that she needs a TOP, which she understands to be an operation under GA with a two-week convalescence. Speak to her about medical TOPs. Explain how the local TOP services are organised.
- Tiki has two specific concerns: arranging time off from work and paying for additional child care.
- You may advise Tiki to tell her employers that she is having a one-off, emergency treatment – this may help to allay their possible concerns about sickness absence. You could offer to provide a sick note, if the hospital does not provide one, if Tiki feels unable to return to work within a week of her TOP. What is written on the sick note could be carefully worded so as not to break Tiki's confidentiality. If Tiki does not want to take sickness absence, she could try

swapping shifts with a colleague to free up some time around the date of her hospital appointment. It may be better to defer the discussion on child care arrangements until firm dates for the TOP are in place.

- Address Tiki's expectations: she expects a referral to the hospital for a TOP. If the doctor feels unable to refer the patient for a TOP because of his or her own personal beliefs, then the doctor should explain this to the patient and make alternative arrangements for the patient's timely referral. It is reasonable to assume that Tiki also expects to be treated with sensitivity and kindness, and for her confidentiality to be respected.

Interpersonal skills:

Good communication with the patient explores the impact of her unwanted pregnancy on her life. This enables the doctor to obtain information about her social circumstances and helps the doctor to contextualise the problem. A willingness to listen and understand may prevent the doctor from allowing his or her own views, values or prejudices to inappropriately influence the patient's decision-making. Therefore, by showing responsiveness to the patient's preferences, feelings and expectations, the doctor and patient work in partnership to develop a shared management plan.

BACKGROUND KNOWLEDGE REQUIRED FOR THIS CASE

The information below is adapted from Marie Stopes patient information leaflet on abortion. www.mariestopes.org.uk/sites/default/files/Abortion%20-%20your%20 questions%20%20answered%20leaflet.pdf

There are two types of treatment for early abortion: medical abortion (abortion pill) or surgical abortion. Medical abortion involves taking hormones in order to pass the pregnancy vaginally – this option is available up to the ninth week of pregnancy. Surgical abortion involves the pregnancy being removed vaginally by an experienced doctor. There is a choice of anaesthetic options with surgical abortion.

Before 9 weeks of pregnancy – early medical abortion: the abortion pill

Up to two visits are necessary (on the same day or on separate days) to complete this treatment. The abortion pill (also called RU486) provides an alternative to having a surgical abortion. Two different drugs are used to cause the pregnancy to pass. Following the second treatment, most women choose to go home while this happens, with 24-hour telephone support from aftercare nurses. Alternatively, women may choose to stay at the termination centre.

Not all women are suitable for medical abortion; it is unsuitable if the patient:

- is over 35 and smokes more than 10 cigarettes a day

- has a suspected ectopic pregnancy
- has a history of heart disease, high blood pressure, liver or kidney disease
- is taking long-term corticosteroids
- has an IUD in place which will not be removed
- has adrenal failure
- is taking anticoagulants or has any haemorrhagic disease or porphyria
- has poorly controlled inflammatory bowel disease.

The failure rate for early medical abortion is between 2 and 3%.

Before 12 weeks of pregnancy – early surgical abortion

At this stage a gentle suction method is used to remove the pregnancy from the uterus. This is a very quick and simple procedure, taking less than five minutes to perform. A general anaesthetic is not necessary.

Between 13 and 19 weeks of pregnancy – surgical abortion

The cervix is dilated. If pregnancy is more than 15 weeks advanced, the cervix is prepared with medication for the procedure. The patient is given the option of conscious sedation or a general anaesthetic.

Between 19 and 24 weeks of pregnancy – later surgical abortion

At this stage of pregnancy the treatment is performed in two separate stages. Stage one involves preparation of the cervix to cause it to gently dilate over a few hours. There is no need to have an anaesthetic for this part of the treatment. The second stage, to complete the abortion, will take place later that day and requires a general anaesthetic.

Relevant literature

RCOG guidelines: **The care of women requesting induced abortion**
Published date: November 2011 – see
http://www.rcog.org.uk/womens-health/clinical-guidance/
care-women-requesting-induced-abortion

Savulescu, J (2006) **Conscientious objection in medicine**, *BMJ*, **332**: 294–297.

Savulescu writes, "A doctor's conscience has little place in the delivery of modern medical care …. If people are not prepared to offer legally permitted, efficient, and beneficial care to a patient because it conflicts with their values, they should not be doctors."

He argues that a service which depends on the values of the treating doctor results in patients shopping among doctors to receive services to which they are entitled. This introduces inefficiency and wastes resources. The less informed patients may fail to receive a service to which they are entitled – this inequity is unjustifiable.

Alternative presentations on this topic

The patient could be a 36-year-old lady who smokes 15 cigarettes per day (or who has a different contra-indication to early medical abortion). Use the information supplied in the Marie Stopes guidance above to construct variations on this case.

CASE 10 Menorrhagia

INFORMATION FOR THE DOCTOR

Name	Alice Bridges
Age	45
Past medical history	Post-natal depression six years ago
Last consultation	Seen by patient's usual GP six months ago and referred to Gynaecology for investigation and treatment of menorrhagia. Excerpt from last consultation:

"Comes to discuss heavy periods again. Mefenamic acid not helping much. Abdominal and pelvic exam essentially normal. Ultrasound scan inconclusive and radiologist advises referral to Gynae as may have small polyp – referral done today."

Hb	10.9g% (13–17)
MCV	86 (83–105)
Cervical smear	normal
BMI	25.6
BP	117/60

INFORMATION FOR THE PATIENT

You are 45-year-old Alice Bridges. Since the birth of your son six years ago, you have had heavy periods. Initially, the time between the periods was shorter (21 days) but over the last two years, your cycle has been more erratic, with the time between periods anything from 21 to 35 days. You have not had a period for seven weeks.

You also experience flushing, sometimes up to three times each day. You feel very warm at night and your sleep is interrupted. You experience mood swings with periodic low moods. Trivial events at work and at home upset you. Once upset, you are tearful and sensitive for the entire day and can't shake it off.

You present with a question for the doctor about your recent attendance at Gynaecology outpatient department. The Gynaecologist told you that she thinks you have an endometrial polyp and need an operation, an endometrial resection, under general anaesthetic (GA) for your heavy periods. But because your periods have stopped for seven weeks, you wonder whether you are in the menopause and no longer require the operation.

Your opening statement is *"I've come to ask for your advice about whether I still need my Gynae operation, doctor"*.

Information to reveal if asked

General information about yourself:

- You are a first-year, mature nursing student. You want to explore your treatment options to gain an understanding of what is happening to you. The Gynaecology consultant said that she thought the pelvic ultrasound showed a polyp, which she was unsuccessful in removing in OPD. She listed you for an endometrial resection under GA. You are not keen on having a GA but will have the operation if it is really needed, but you think you have menopausal symptoms and so your periods should end soon, making the operation redundant.

- You are doing well with your nursing studies; you are busy juggling home and nursing-student demands but you enjoy these challenges.

Further details about your condition:

- The proposed scheduling of the operation would not cause problems at home or work.
- You do not think that you are pregnant; you use barrier contraception.
- You do not want a Mirena IUS; this was discussed with the Gynaecology consultant.
- You do not have a significant family history.

Your ideas:

> If you have not bled for 7 weeks, are you in the menopause? Should you go through with this operation? You would prefer not to have any interventions (operation or HRT) unless the benefit outweighs the risks. You have coped with heavy periods but the disturbed mood and interrupted sleep are taking their toll.

Your concerns:

> If your periods are going to stop soon with the menopause, is this operation now redundant? If you need the operation, how much time off are you likely to need? Will you be able to look after your son, or should your husband take a few days off work?

Your expectations:

> You want this doctor's advice on the endometrial resection and you also want advice on treatments for the menopause. You prefer natural remedies because you heard about HRT increasing your risk of breast cancer, but you would like to read about HRT before making any treatment choices.

Medical history

> You are in good general health; use condoms reliably and are not on long-term medication. You do not have a history of gallstones, migraines or DVT.

Social history

> You have a six-year-old son and your family is complete. Your husband has been very supportive but he is concerned about your mood swings. There have not been any specific problems at home or work as yet.

Information to reveal if examined

> You are not anxious or depressed.

SUGGESTED APPROACH TO THE CONSULTATION

Targeted history taking:

- When did she see the consultant and what was discussed in OPD? You have not received a copy of the hospital letter as yet.

- What did she understand by the word 'polyp'?

- Why does she think it is important to remove the polyp?

- Does she have any concerns about the operation or a GA or the recovery time?

- What are the symptoms causing the greatest distress at present?

- What does she think she has?

- Does she think she is menopausal?

- What treatments for menopausal symptoms is she aware of?

- Is her mind made up about natural therapies or is she willing to consider the risks and benefits of HRT/SSRIs?

Targeted examination:

- Examination is not required in this case.

Clinical management:

- Address the patient's ideas – that seven weeks of amenorrhoea, with her recent irregular periods and peri-menopausal symptoms may mean that she is unlikely to get further heavy bleeding, but periods could fluctuate during this period – they are unpredictable.

- Fulfil her expectations for advice about the polyp and treatments for peri-menopausal symptoms: despite the seven-week history of amenorrhoea, histological evaluation of the polyp is needed, either by endometrial resection or by hysteroscopy. Regarding the endometrial resection, you could say that this procedure is both diagnostic (the entire endometrium is available for histological evaluation) and therapeutic (as a treatment for menorrhagia). In contrast, hysteroscopy with endometrial biopsy would be diagnostic only. An IUS can be inserted at the time of endometrial resection or hysteroscopy: this treats the menorrhagia and also gives endometrial protection if oestrogen-only HRT is used. Oestrogen-only HRT may have a lower risk of breast cancer than oral combination HRT.

- You need to briefly discuss the risks and benefits of HRT, or signpost the patient to appropriate balanced information so that she can be better informed before making a choice about whether or not to start HRT.

Interpersonal skills:

Good communication with the patient:

- demonstrates a respect for her curiosity as a nursing student.

- demonstrates a respect for the limitations of hospital systems within which consultant colleagues work. It would be easy to make disparaging comments about the relative lateness of the discharge letter.

- shows responsiveness to the patient's preferences, feelings and expectations for further information on surgery and HRT.

- communicates the relevant information in a manner that is understandable to the patient, without slipping into jargon and without patronising the patient.

Therefore, it results in addressing the patient's expectations appropriately.

BACKGROUND KNOWLEDGE REQUIRED FOR THIS CASE

Pitkin, J (2007) **Dysfunctional uterine bleeding**, *BMJ*, **334**: 1110–1111.

- Irregular heavy bleeding in women in their late 40s is often attributed to starting the menopause, but still needs investigation. Endometrial carcinoma can occur in the late 40s. About 6% of endometrial cancers can occur with heavy regular bleeds.

- Confirm that menorrhagia has been present for several menstrual cycles.

- **Investigation**: A full blood count is needed; endocrine investigations such as thyroid function tests are not routinely necessary. An endometrial biopsy is not required in the initial assessment of menorrhagia.

- **Treatment**: Tranexamic acid and mefenamic acid are effective treatments for reducing heavy menstrual blood loss, even in women who have an intrauterine contraceptive device *in situ*. Combined oral contraceptives, a progestogen-releasing intrauterine device, or other long-acting progestogens can reduce menstrual blood loss.

Alternative presentations on this topic:

The patient could present with previously uninvestigated heavy menstrual bleeding or wanting information about the Mirena IUS as a treatment option. If so, how would she present and what would be the appropriate GP management? Use the information supplied below to construct variations on this case.

NICE guidelines [CG44] Published date: January 2007

Heavy menstrual bleeding (HMB) should be defined as excessive menstrual blood loss which interferes with the woman's physical, emotional, social and material quality of life, and which can occur alone or in combination with other symptoms. Any interventions should aim to improve quality of life measures.

History taking, examination and investigations

If appropriate, a biopsy should be taken to exclude endometrial cancer or atypical hyperplasia. Indications for a biopsy include, for example, persistent intermenstrual bleeding, and in women aged 45 and over, treatment failure or ineffective treatment.

Ultrasound is the first-line diagnostic tool for identifying structural abnormalities.

Education and information provision

A woman with HMB referred to specialist care should be given information before her outpatient appointment.

Pharmaceutical treatment

If history and investigations indicate that pharmaceutical treatment is appropriate and either hormonal or non-hormonal treatments are acceptable, treatments should be considered in the following order:

1. Levonorgestrel-releasing intrauterine system (LNG-IUS) provided long-term (at least 12 months) use is anticipated
2. Tranexamic acid or non-steroidal anti-inflammatory drugs (NSAIDs) or combined oral contraceptives (COCs)
3. Norethisterone (15mg) daily from days 5 to 26 of the menstrual cycle, or injected long-acting progestogens.

If hormonal treatments are not acceptable to the woman, then either tranexamic acid or NSAIDs can be used.

Non-hysterectomy surgery

In women with HMB alone, with uterus no bigger than a 10-week pregnancy, endometrial ablation should be considered preferable to hysterectomy.

Hysterectomy

Taking into account the need for individual assessment, the route of hysterectomy should be considered in the following order: first line vaginal; second line abdominal.

CASE 11 **Hypothyroidism**

INFORMATION FOR THE DOCTOR

Name	David Fields
Age	41
Social and family history	Married, two children
Past medical history	• Subclinical hypothyroidism 5 months ago • Morton's neuroma 5 years ago • Wry neck 8 years ago • Diarrhoea on diclofenac
Current medication	Levothyroxine 75mcg once daily
Blood tests TSH 8 months ago TSH* 5 months ago TSH 1 month ago	*Recent blood tests* 4.99 (0.35–5.5) 7.89 (0.35–5.5) and Free T$_4$ within normal range 3.72 (0.35–5.5)
U&Es, LFTs and FBC 8 months ago – within normal limits	
Plasma fasting glucose	5.1mmol/L (3.65–5.5)
Weight Height BMI BP	96kg 177cm 30.6 136/84

INFORMATION FOR THE PATIENT

You are David Fields, a 41-year-old infrastructure manager for a multinational. You were diagnosed with hypothyroidism 5 months ago and have been taking thyroxine 75mcg daily. Your TSH from a month ago was 3.72, which you understand to be normal, but you are still tired and want to know if you can increase your levothyroxine dose.

The 75mcg of levothyroxine was a 'tester' dose, which you were keen to take, hoping it would help with your tiredness. There was difficulty in making the diagnosis of hypothyroidism – the first TSH was normal, the second TSH was 7.89. Because your usual doctor wasn't absolutely sure of the diagnosis, he put you on thyroxine 75mcg five months ago and rechecked the TSH last month when it was 3.72. You do not have any side-effects from the medication but you remain tired.

By tired, you mean physical and mental lethargy – 'your get up and go has got up and gone'. You don't feel like you are coming down with something. You have been tired for eighteen months, since prior to the diagnosis of hypothyroidism. Once the diagnosis was made, and tests done at your insistence, and you started levothyroxine tablets, you hoped that the tiredness would lift. You are 'tired all the time'. You wake up feeling as if you could go right back to sleep. In the evenings, you slump in your chair and nod off in front of the TV. You go to bed at 9.30pm and wake up at 5.30am and despite the eight hours of uninterrupted sleep, you still feel tired.

You do not have any other symptoms of hypothyroidism. If asked specifically, you do not have memory problems, constipation or weight gain. Your hair is thinning slightly, but you assumed that is normal for your age. You are irritable and you worry about money, children and your job but you do not feel more stressed than usual. You don't feel depressed or low or hopeless.

There are current home and work stresses; you say 'it has been a bad month'. Your 16-year-old daughter is doing GCSEs at the moment. Unlike your wife, you worry whether she is revising enough. Your job as an infrastructure manager changed recently – instead of remotely reviewing the budget for various building and maintenance jobs, you now have to visit sites scattered throughout the region. This involves approximately eight additional hours of driving each week, four on Monday and four on Wednesday. This also makes coming to the surgery on those days tricky, hence your difficulty in seeing your usual GP. The commuting, especially on the M4, is challenging. You have not fallen asleep at the wheel but you worry about this. You do not think that you are stressed by the changes at work – 'this tiredness is not in my head'.

You present to the doctor hoping to increase your levothyroxine dose to help with your tiredness. Your opening statement is *"I think I may need a higher dose of thyroxine to help shift my tiredness"*.

Information to reveal if asked

General information about yourself:

- As an infrastructure manager, your usual commute is 30 minutes, but longer if you visit various regional sites.
- Your wife did not attend university. She works part-time as an admin assistant.
- Your daughter, you believe, is capable of going to University but seems distracted by fashion, hair and boys at present. When you try to be stern about work, your wife says you are being too hard on her.
- You tend to socialise with your wife's friends at weekends.
- You take your son to football and cricket practice and meet up with other dads there.
- You are in good health usually. You are a non-smoker. You drink four to six beers over the weekend.
- Nobody in your family has thyroid disease.

Further details about your condition:

- You do not take over-the-counter medication.
- You have not lost weight nor had a change in appetite.
- Your thirst, urination, and bowel habits have not changed.
- Your libido has decreased but you do not have problems with erections.
- Your wife has not complained that you snore loudly or that you 'stop breathing' for short periods in your sleep.
- Your relationship with your wife is 'fine'.
- You enjoy your work and you are proud of what you have achieved. The job has changed and you have had to change with it. You do not enjoy the extra driving but you do enjoy the variation in the working week the off-site work has brought.

Your ideas:

- You think that your tiredness is due to a thyroid problem. If the first set of tests didn't pick up the problem, and the bloods only showed a problem when retested, you think that the thyroid tests are sometimes unreliable.
- You think a higher dose of tablets should be OK but you didn't want to increase the medication without checking, in case you overdosed. The patient leaflet was a bit scary so you wanted to discuss the change in dosage with the doctor first.

- If the doctor wants to order more blood tests or refer you, you'd like to know why. Is the doctor concerned about a more serious cause for your tiredness?
- You don't think you are depressed or anxious.
- You don't think exercising is going to make you feel less tired. Doctors tell everyone to eat five a day and exercise more, don't they?

Your concerns:

- You are worried about falling asleep at the wheel. This has not happened but you worry about the level of concentration your driving requires. These long commuting days are the days on which you feel most tired. You feel least tired on the weekend.

Your expectations:

- You expect to be advised about increasing your dose of levothyroxine.
- You expect to be advised on when you should next get a blood test.
- You expect some advice on what to do if the higher dose of levothyroxine does not help your tiredness.

Medical history

You are overweight and have been so for years, but you do not consider yourself to be unhealthy. You do not have side-effects from levothyroxine.

Social history

You are happily married. You get on better with your 10-year-old son than with your 16-year-old daughter at present. She is in a 'difficult phase'. You enjoy your current social life.

Information to reveal if examined

If the doctor asks to examine your thyroid gland, hand him/her a card saying "no goitre palpated".

SUGGESTED APPROACH TO THE CONSULTATION

Targeted history taking:

- What does he mean by tiredness? Is he describing mental or physical fatigue, lethargy or general malaise?

- For how long has he been tired? Did it follow an illness (sore throat)? Is the tiredness getting worse? What could he do before that he cannot do now?

- When is he tired? Is he more tired at certain times of day, certain days of the week?

- When does he take his medication? Is he compliant?

- Why was he put on this dose of thyroxine?

- Does he have other symptoms of hypothyroidism, such as weight gain, constipation, hoarse voice or dry skin and hair?

- What job does he do?

- Could there be other reasons for his tiredness, such as poor quality and quantity of sleep, changes at home or at work, stress?

- What are his expectations of this consultation: an exploration of the possible causes of tiredness, further blood tests, a change in his medication, referral to an endocrinologist, time off work?

- What is his general health like – have other causes of tiredness been excluded?

- Does anyone in his family have hypothyroidism and what has their experience of the illness been?

Targeted examination:

- A targeted physical examination of the thyroid is required to assess whether a goitre is present. See http://www.youtube.com/watch?v=JYb-io13fOA for a demonstration on how to examine the thyroid gland.

Clinical management:

- Explore the possible causes of tiredness. If he is not keen to explore psychological issues at present and if you assess that he is not depressed, then try to maintain rapport and address his ideas about inadequately treated subclinical hypothyroidism being the cause of his tiredness.

- Discuss the significance of the negative examination findings. Adult patients with serum TSH <10mIU/L are treated if (1) symptomatic; (2) have infertility/are pregnant; (3) have a goitre or (4) have positive anti-thyroid peroxidase (TPO) antibodies. Except for the tiredness, he does not have any other symptoms of hypothyroidism. As your examination today did not reveal a goitre, his TPO antibodies need to be checked and/or levothyroxine be tried at a full replacement dose for a trial period (usually 3–6 months) before the diagnosis is reconsidered.

- His idea that his dose of thyroxine is too low may certainly be valid. Most 75kg men without IHD under 60 years of age need approximately 125mcg levothyroxine daily (60kg women need 100mcg daily); starting at full replacement dose and titrating (based on 8–12 week TSH measurements) to reach a TSH of 0.4 to 2.5mU/L.

- Discuss possible options: increasing the dose of thyroxine and review, perhaps with a blood test, in 8–12 weeks; or stay on the same dose but address issues at work and home that could be contributing to his tiredness.

- Address the patient's concerns and expectations: he is concerned about falling asleep at the wheel and expects that his tiredness will improve once he takes a higher dose. You advise him of what is an appropriate higher dose and issue the medication. However, it is important to exclude sleep apnoea (red flag).

- Explain how to take the medication (are you issuing 100mcg tablets, 50mcg or 25mcg tablets?). Encourage compliance with the medication. He could take the medication in the morning or at night if he does not eat late at night. If he is forgetful, and seeing that he does not have IHD or AF, he could take seven times the daily dose once a week.

- Safety-net: advise him of when you would next like to review him and under what circumstances he should return early for reassessment. If you are organising blood tests, consider getting TFTs, TPO antibodies, lipids and perhaps bloods to exclude coeliac disease, as the latter was not ruled out in the original diagnostic sieve. Although there is an association with hypothyroidism and dyslipidaemia, the relationship of subclinical hypothyroidism with CV disease is less clear. However, it may be useful to assess, stratify and treat CV risk so an offer of lipid screening is not unreasonable.

Interpersonal skills:

This case tests the doctor's ability to review a diagnosis and demonstrate therapeutic skills. The patient is convinced that he has a physical cause for his tiredness: one blood test showed subclinical hypothyroidism but the patient does not seem to be responding as expected to treatment with levothyroxine. Either a longer trial of treatment with a higher dose of medication is needed (this is the patient's agenda) or the diagnosis needs review (doctor's agenda). The skilful doctor reviews the issue systematically and holistically, negotiates the conflicting agendas and works in partnership with the patient. Acknowledging the validity of the patient's beliefs creates rapport and enables the development of an effectual therapeutic relationship.

The poor communicator is unable to devise a safe management plan that is responsive to the patient's health beliefs and concerns. Instead, he or she adopts a rigid approach and fails to forge a useful therapeutic alliance with the patient.

BACKGROUND KNOWLEDGE REQUIRED FOR THIS CASE

The diagnosis and management of primary hypothyroidism; Royal College of Physicians and others (June 2011).

Treatment of sub-clinical hypothyroidism

(a) Sub-clinical hypothyroidism is defined as being present in a patient when the TSH is above the upper limit of the reference range (but usually less than 10mU/L) and free T_4 levels are within the reference range.

(b) Some patients with sub-clinical hypothyroidism, particularly those whose TSH level is greater than 10mU/L, may benefit from treatment with levothyroxine in the same way as for clinical hypothyroidism, as indicated in national guidelines (British Thyroid Association, The Association for Clinical Biochemistry, British Thyroid Foundation. *UK guidelines for the use of thyroid function tests*. London, BTA/ACB/BTF: 2006.) www.acb.org.uk/docs/TFTguidelinefinal.pdf

Treatment of primary hypothyroidism

(a) The aim of the treatment of hypothyroidism is to render the patient back to the normal or 'euthyroid' state.

(b) When a sufficient dose of thyroid treatment is given to lower the TSH to within the normal range (reference range) for the test method used, patients usually recover from their symptoms of hypothyroidism.

(c) Fine-tuning of TSH levels inside the reference range may be needed for individual patients.

(d) Patients with continuing symptoms after appropriate thyroxine treatment should be further investigated to diagnose and treat the cause.

Moncrieff, G and Fletcher, J (2007) **Tiredness,** *BMJ*, **334**: 1221.

This 10-minute consultation article suggests that patients who present with tiredness consult for many reasons:

- It may be a symptom of physical disease, such as hypothyroidism, autoimmune disease, liver or kidney disease, or malignancy.

- It may be a symptom of depression or a response to the stresses of life circumstances.

- It may be a tester symptom, where it is offered as an initial symptom to see whether the doctor is sympathetic and interested, before the main, perhaps sensitive, agenda is revealed. 'Patients may consider tiredness to be a more legitimate symptom to bring to a doctor than, say, unhappiness.'

How should doctors deal with their patients' unhappiness? One approach is to employ active listening skills and allow the patient to tell their story.

Telling illness stories

From http://www.aissg.org/articles/TELLING.HTM:

'Illness stories are therapeutic for *tellers* who have a real opportunity to be heard and to hear themselves. As they tell and retell their story they can unravel the truth of their own experience of illness and begin to adjust to the person they have become. From this position they can begin to uncover the person they could become. Telling their story has given them the opportunity to step outside of themselves and witness who they are. This dis-identification allows new possibilities to emerge.'

Active listening skills – from: http://www.holisticlocal.co.uk/articles/view/293/The+Therapeutic+Relationship:

"What are the skills required by the practitioner to instate a strong therapeutic relationship that can beget great benefit for patients?....

The therapeutic skills [are]:

- Unconditional Acceptance
- Empathy
- Attending and Listening
- Open Questioning
- Reflection
- Silence
- Physical and Behavioural Techniques
- Concreteness
- Professionalism
- Warmth and Being Genuine"

CASE 12 Calf pain

INFORMATION FOR THE DOCTOR

Name	James Prentiss
Age	25
Social and family history	Unmarried, no children
Past medical history	• Patella tendinopathy 2 years ago • Thoracic back pain (mechanical) 3 years ago • Seborrhoeic dermatitis 8 years ago

The medical record of his **last medical entry** two weeks ago reads:

"Patient discharged from fracture clinic. Was training with bobsleigh team in Hamburg 10 weeks ago when fell heavily while getting into bobsleigh. Sustained an undisplaced fracture of his R 4th MT. Fracture clinic removed aircast boot after 6 weeks and advised patient to mobilise in supportive boots for a month. Comes today for fit-note. Engineer and feels ready to move out of office-based work in repair bay work – can kneel and work at heights – note issued."

Current medication	Ibuprofen 400mg TDS, as needed
Clinical values BP Weight Height BMI	 134/84 100kg 180cm 30.7

INFORMATION FOR THE PATIENT

You are James Prentiss, a 29-year-old engineer, who has come to discuss the problems you experience with your right foot and calf. You fractured your R 4th MT 10 weeks ago in bobsleigh training; had a CT in Germany; were placed in a plaster cast that was cut down the middle; put on blood thinning injections and sent home. In your local hospital, they X-rayed you; stopped the injections and changed you into an aircast boot. The fracture clinic doctor undertook telephone follow-up at 5 weeks and told you to remove the aircast boot and wear Hi-Tec type boots for 4 weeks.

Two weeks ago, when you changed from wearing boots to wearing shoes and trainers, you developed pain over the top of your right foot, stretching from the area of the fracture over the top of the foot. Four weeks ago, you also developed right calf swelling, so much so that you have worn rugby skins to compress the swelling. If you don't wear rugby skins, you can press on the calf swelling and it leaves an indentation. The physiotherapist noticed this a week ago. She thought you may need to return to the fracture clinic to check that the fracture has healed properly.

You think that the MT fracture has not healed properly and would like to be referred back to fracture clinic for an X-ray. Your opening statement is *"I'm really bothered by this foot pain".*

Information to reveal if asked

General information about yourself:

- You are an engineer at the local branch of a train maintenance company.

- You sustained your injury during high level bobsleigh training. You are trying to get into the national team.

Further details about your condition:

- If specifically asked about the foot pain, it is a dull ache (2/10) that gets worse at the end of the day (4/10). You were much better in boots but when you switched to shoes, the pain increased and despite taking paracetamol and ibuprofen, it has persisted. It is worse if you stand for long periods. Your physiotherapist has not started you on a run/walk programme as yet, so you don't know how running would impact the pain.

- If asked about the swelling, it has been there since the plaster cast was removed and the airboot fitted. You were sent home from Hamburg on Fragmin injections but the fracture clinic doctor told you to stop the injections when he removed the plaster and put you in an aircast boot. You thought the initial swelling was because you were unable to keep your foot up during the flight home. Now you think that because you don't exercise the R calf as much, you have not been able to get rid of the swelling. You wonder if the calf muscle is torn and swollen.

- You do not have any chest pain or shortness of breath.

- You are usually fit and healthy.

Your ideas:

- You think that you may have done too much too soon and perhaps you inadvertently re-injured the healing fracture.

- You had a very nasty fall and think that you trapped the R foot under the bobsleigh and twisted, so you may have torn the calf muscle, hence the swelling.

Your concerns:

- You are worried that you have problems with fracture healing. If you don't get back to running soon, you will miss this winter's training.

Your expectations:

- You expect to be referred back to fracture clinic or at least, get an X-ray of the R foot.

Medical history

Physically, you are in good general health, and do not have heartburn, ulcers or bleeding problems.

Social history

You are training hard to compete at bobsleigh. You watch what you eat. You do not smoke. You occasionally drink alcohol when not in active training.

Information to reveal if examined

Show a picture: http://www.gponline.com/red-flag-symptoms-swollen-calf/haematology/article/1013798

Only the R lateral calf near the fibula head is tender.

The R leg is swollen to mid thigh.

The R calf is 5cm larger than the left.

There is pitting oedema of the R calf.

SUGGESTED APPROACH TO THE CONSULTATION

Targeted history taking:

- Take a detailed history of James's symptoms:
  - calf pain: onset, intensity, aggravating and relieving factors, radiation, associated symptoms
  - calf swelling
- Explore James's ideas about why the pain may have suddenly intensified and why the swelling has been so extensive.
- He stated his concerns at the outset. Explore his fears about a delayed return to competitive bobsleigh.
- Explore his expectations – how does he want the foot pain investigated?
- Explore the calf swelling in greater detail – take a good history to assess the likelihood of DVT or PE.

Targeted examination:

- Perform an examination of the foot and calf for tenderness, swelling, change in skin colour and temperature, and range of movement of foot.
- Use the examination findings to complete a Wells' score.

Clinical management:

- Complete a Wells' score:

Clinical feature	Points	Patient score
Active cancer (treatment ongoing, within 6 months, or palliative)	1	
Paralysis, paresis or recent plaster immobilisation of the lower extremities	1	1
Recently bedridden for 3 days or more or major surgery within 12 weeks requiring general or regional anaesthesia	1	
Localised tenderness along the distribution of the deep venous system	1	
Entire leg swollen	1	1
Calf swelling at least 3 cm larger than asymptomatic side	1	1
Pitting oedema confined to the symptomatic leg	1	1
Collateral superficial veins (non-varicose)	1	
Previously documented DVT	1	
An alternative diagnosis is at least as likely as DVT	−2	−2
Clinical probability simplified score		
DVT *likely*	2 points or more	2
DVT *unlikely*	1 point or less	

- Discuss a possible diagnosis of DVT as an explanation of calf swelling and possible delayed union or foot bio-mechanical issues as an explanation for the R foot pain.

- Discuss the treatment options – James needs to have an ultrasound scan within 4 hours if possible. You need to contact the DVT clinic to arrange this. If the scan is delayed by more than 4 hours, you need to organise a blood test for d-dimers and prescribe rivaroxaban 15mg BD until the scan appointment.

- Address James's ideas: that an X-ray is needed. The foot pain may be due to delayed fracture healing so you will arrange follow-up in fracture clinic. Until then, he could return to wearing boots if this was more comfortable than shoes.

- Address the patient's concerns about returning to competitive sport. *"I think we need the results of the DVT scan and the foot X-ray before we can discuss the effect on your sport. What do you think?"*

- Address the patient's expectations: refer to DVT clinic and arrange for fracture clinic follow-up.

- Confirm his understanding of DVT and provide sufficient information about the condition, its investigation and treatment options – consider a patient information leaflet.

- Arrange suitable follow-up after his appointments at DVT and fracture clinic.

Interpersonal skills:

This case tests the doctor's ability to explore a presenting problem more deeply, eliciting the presence of 'red flags' resulting in the diagnosis of a lower limb complication, namely DVT. It also tests the doctor's ability to prioritise treatment agendas: referral to DVT clinic takes precedence. The doctor's interpersonal skills are demonstrated in negotiating agendas and arranging suitable follow-up to address issues that had to be parked today.

Good communication with the patient:

- encourages the patient to explore his symptoms through the skilful use of open questions: *"I'm really interested in this calf swelling – tell me more. What do you think is causing it?"*

- makes statements to widen the patient's agenda: *"Based on your history and examination findings, your Wells' score shows a high likelihood of DVT – a clot in the leg veins. What is your understanding of a clot in the leg? Do you know anyone who had treatment for this?"*

- builds trust through reflective listening: *"It sounds like there are issues here about returning to competitive sport. Let's get the results from DVT clinic and fracture clinic, then meet again to discuss a plan going forward. How does that sound?"*

- encourages reflection: *"Look, you came in thinking you might need a foot X-ray and here I am sending you for an urgent DVT scan. How do you feel about this?"*

Poor communication with the patient:

- addresses the patient's agenda only and does not explore the calf swelling (the red flag).

- fails to discuss what a DVT is and explain why urgent diagnosis and treatment is needed. Without this information, the patient is not empowered to amend their concerns and expectations.

- is prescriptive in his or her management: *"You need a scan. Never mind about your foot and this bobsleigh competition – that's the least of your worries."*

BACKGROUND KNOWLEDGE REQUIRED FOR THIS CASE

NICE guidelines (2012)(CG 144)

Venous thromboembolic diseases: the management of venous thromboembolic diseases and the role of thrombophilia testing. http://www.nice.org.uk/guidance/cg144/chapter/guidance

Relevant literature

For a DVT clinic protocol, see http://oxford-haematology.org.uk/sites/default/files/Outpatient%20DVT%20protocols.pdf

The following patients may need referral to alternative services, such as specialised obstetric/haematology or medical teams:

- Pregnancy
- Suspected upper limb DVT
- In-patients (unless investigation complete and being discharged)
- Unable to transfer from chair to chair by self
- Primary diagnosis of pulmonary embolism
- >180kg
- Active bleeding
- Known to be at increased risk of bleeding, e.g.
  - active peptic ulceration
  - liver disease (PT >18 secs)
  - renal insufficiency: creatinine >200μmol/L with unknown eGFR or
  - eGFR <20mL/min/1.73m^2 (eGFR calculator at www.renal.org/egfrcalc)
  - uncontrolled hypertension (>200/110mmHg)
  - recent (<1/12) eye or CNS surgery
  - recent (<1/12) haemorrhagic stroke

CASE 13 Eczema

INFORMATION FOR THE DOCTOR

You are a doctor in surgery. You are visited by Caroline Jacobs and her daughter Ellen.

Name	Ellen Jacobs
Age	2
Social and family history	Only child, parents aged 36 and 33
Past medical history	• Treated for an 'eczema flare' 4 weeks ago with antibiotics and Eumovate • Seen by a community dermatology nurse 9 months ago – atopic eczema
Repeat medication	• Dermol cream 500mg apply thrice daily • Aveeno at night • Hydrocortisone as required or once daily for 5–7 days • Dermol 600 bath emollient – use daily in bath

INFORMATION FOR THE PATIENT

You are Caroline Jacobs, 36-year-old mother of Ellen, a 2-year-old who has had eczema practically since birth. You are worried about the severity of your daughter's eczema. You are seeing the doctor today because you require a repeat prescription for Ellen's medication and a set of emollients for nursery. You also want to talk to the doctor about a new treatment for eczema. You recently attended a dinner party where one of the other guests, a health visitor, spoke to you about a new treatment, an 'anti-cancer' cream for eczema.

Ellen's eczema flared last month. You think it was because nursery are not applying the cream regularly – they use one tub in the same time as it takes you to go through three tubs. You have had to put Ellen in nursery as you have returned to work part-time as an administrator. You feel guilty about delegating her care to nursery. Ellen was very uncomfortable last month when her eczema flared; she scratched herself so badly at night that she bled. You took two days off work, kept Ellen at home and applied the creams properly. Her skin improved. You worry that the 'sub-standard' care she gets at nursery will aggravate her eczema and you wonder if other things such as changing Ellen's diet may help. When you mentioned your concerns to your mother-in-law, she was very keen to take Ellen to her homeopath who worked 'miracles' with her friend's problematic skin.

You present to the doctor expecting to discuss Ellen's repeat prescription and to ask if anything else, such as dietary changes or homeopathy, should be trialled.

Information to reveal if asked

General information about yourself and Ellen:

- You have found returning to work challenging but good. You feel guilty about not being there for Ellen, especially when she is miserable with her eczema flares.

- You have spoken to nursery about applying the emollients regularly. While they agree with you, you suspect because of the under-utilisation of the creams, that they are not as diligent as you. They also encourage Ellen to finger paint, play in the sandpit and use play dough. While you are not unhappy with this, you wish they would wash Ellen more carefully after these activities and apply the creams after each wash.

- You had an uneventful pregnancy and delivery with Ellen.

- You have hayfever but nobody in your family or your husband's family has eczema or asthma.

Further details about Ellen's condition:

- Ellen has had eczema from birth. She had dry patches of skin around the corners of her mouth, in the neck creases and on her elbows and knees. Now, she has patches on her elbows and knees. When the patches get bigger, redder and itchy, Ellen becomes unhappy, irritable, scratches more and has disturbed sleep. With regular emollient use, these flares have become irregular; the last occurred last month and the one before that, 3 months ago.

- If specifically asked, you discuss that you have not noticed that anything in particular (except very hot, sticky weather) triggers Ellen's flares. She does not react to particular foods or lotions or washing powders or animals. She is growing well. She does not have colic, vomiting or diarrhoea.
- Ellen likes nursery.

Your ideas:

- You think that Ellen's creams work, if only nursery would apply them appropriately.
- You think steroid creams are useful. When you apply the steroid cream, Ellen scratches a lot less and sleeps well. However, you are curious about a steroid sparing cream, but concerned about it being described as an anti-cancer cream. You would like some information.
- If the doctor offers to prescribe the anti-cancer cream, such as tacrolimus or pimecrolimus, you are a bit hesitant and want to know about possible side-effects.
- If you become comfortable with the doctor's consultation manner, you reveal that you think homeopathy 'is a load of drivel'. You think that your mother-in-law does not approve of your returning to work and you perceive her wish to take Ellen to a homeopath as indirect criticism of your child-raising.

Your concerns:

- You are worried about Ellen's eczema deteriorating because nursery are not diligent about cream application.

Your expectations:

- You expect to get a repeat prescription for Ellen's medication, information about anti-cancer creams for eczema, ideas about what to do about nursery and an opinion on dietary changes and homeopathy for eczema.

Medical history

Ellen was seen more than a year ago by the Paediatric Community Nurse who advised wet dressings for a short period.

Social history

You are happily married. You are not sure if you want to have a second child.

Information to reveal if examined

Examination is not necessary.

SUGGESTED APPROACH TO THE CONSULTATION

Targeted history taking:

- What does Ellen's skin look like now – where does she have dry patches, how big, how severe?

- What is her response to the current treatment regime? Are there any problems with the medication, including any side-effects?

- Does Mrs Jacobs think that something could be triggering 'flares' – any allergens or irritants?

- Is Ellen growing well? Is there associated hayfever or asthma? Does Ellen have any bowel symptoms to suggest an associated food allergy?

- How is the eczema affecting Ellen and the family?

- What are Mrs Jacobs' concerns? Is she worried about possible causes for the last flare; the possibility that the current medication regime is inadequate; cream application?

- What are her expectations: repeat prescription; a change to the prescription; signposting to information about tacrolimus or pimecrolimus; dietary advice?

- Is she prepared to revisit nursery and does she require any help with getting the nursery staff on board?

- Is she prepared to step up and step down medication? Does she know how and when to do this?

Targeted examination:

- This case does not require the candidate to perform a targeted physical examination.

Clinical management:

- Discuss the diagnosis and severity. Based on Mrs Jacob's description, it does sound like Ellen has atopic eczema. Usually this is mild, with areas of dry, sometimes red skin, infrequent itching with little effect on daytime activities and sleep. However, in a 'flare' she has moderately severe eczema, with dry red skin, frequent itching, disturbed sleep and daytime irritability.

- Discuss the treatment of mild and moderate eczema, how to recognise a flare, how to step treatment up and down and how to identify possible triggers.

- Address the patient's ideas and discuss what could have triggered the most recent flare. Mrs Jacobs' idea that it was triggered by nursery not applying the emollients regularly, and possibly washing with soap rather than soap substitutes, is most likely correct. It is difficult to suspect a food trigger – Ellen has not had bowel symptoms, is growing well and her eczema previously responded well to her medication.

- Discuss topical tacrolimus and pimecrolimus; both can be used as second-line treatments in a 2-year-old, when steroids do not adequately control symptoms.
- Address the patient's concerns about nursery. Discuss what help Mrs Jacobs needs with regard to nursery. Most children with atopic eczema require 250 to 500g of emollients per week, so one 500g tub lasting 3 weeks at nursery rather points to under-use. It may be that Mrs Jacobs simply required this information from you before talking to the nursery nurses.
- Address the patient's expectations about a repeat prescription. This includes a discussion on how emollients and steroids are applied – see NICE CG57 for information on types of emollients and steroids as well as quantity, timing, process of application, stepping up, etc.
- Discuss how complementary therapies such as homeopathy for the management of atopic eczema have not yet been adequately assessed in clinical studies.
- Confirm Mrs Jacobs' understanding of treatment:
  - how much of the treatments to use
  - how often to apply treatments
  - when and how to step treatment up or down
  - how to treat infected atopic eczema.
- Consider follow-up with Ellen, to examine her skin and its response to the current prescription regime and to consider if topical tacrolimus and pimecrolimus is needed.

Interpersonal skills:

This case primarily tests two important skills:

1. The doctor's ability to assess the impact of a chronic illness on the patient and his or her family, that is, to undertake a *holistic* assessment, and
2. The doctor's ability to discuss a step-wise approach to managing that chronic illness: recognising triggers, stepping up and stepping down.

Good communication with the patient:

- explores what the patient already knows and gives the patient new information that builds on existing ideas. For example, Mrs Jacobs already knows what is mild eczema in Ellen, and what constitutes a 'flare' or moderately severe eczema. This leads quite neatly into a discussion about what could trigger a flare, what medication can be used to treat a flare, the difference between mild and moderate potency corticosteroids, and when stepping up to topical tacrolimus and pimecrolimus may be needed.

- explores the illness holistically. By the end of data-gathering, the doctor understands the impact of the illness on the child's (and parents') everyday activities, sleep and psychosocial wellbeing and is able to offer targeted support.

- good prescribing behaviour involves discussing how to apply the emollients and steroids.

BACKGROUND KNOWLEDGE REQUIRED FOR THIS CASE

NICE guidelines [CG57] (Dec 2007), **Atopic eczema in children: Management of atopic eczema in children from birth up to the age of 12 years.**

Table 13.1 Holistic assessment

Skin/physical severity		Impact on quality of life and psychosocial wellbeing	
Clear	Normal skin, no evidence of active atopic eczema	None	No impact on quality of life
Mild	Areas of dry skin, infrequent itching (with or without small areas of redness)	Mild	Little impact on everyday activities, sleep and psychosocial wellbeing
Moderate	Areas of dry skin, frequent itching, redness (with or without excoriation and localised skin thickening)	Moderate	Moderate impact on everyday activities and psychosocial wellbeing, frequently disturbed sleep
Severe	Widespread areas of dry skin, incessant itching, redness (with or without excoriation, extensive skin thickening, bleeding, oozing, cracking and alteration of pigmentation)	Severe	Severe limitation of everyday activities and psychosocial functioning, nightly loss of sleep

Healthcare professionals should consider a diagnosis of food allergy in children with atopic eczema who:

- have reacted previously to a food with immediate symptoms, or
- in infants and young children with moderate or severe atopic eczema that has not been controlled by optimum management, particularly if associated with gut dysmotility (colic, vomiting, altered bowel habit) or failure to thrive.

Healthcare professionals should reassure children with mild atopic eczema and their parents or carers that most children with mild atopic eczema do not need to have tests for allergies.

Table 13.2 Treatment options

Mild atopic eczema	Moderate atopic eczema	Severe atopic eczema
Emollients	Emollients	Emollients
Mild potency topical corticosteroids	Moderate potency topical corticosteroids	Potent topical corticosteroids
	Topical calcineurin inhibitors	Topical calcineurin inhibitors
	Bandages	Bandages
		Phototherapy
		Systemic therapy

Healthcare professionals should offer children with atopic eczema and their parents or carers information on how to recognise flares of atopic eczema (increased dryness, itching, redness, swelling and general irritability). They should give clear instructions on how to manage flares according to the stepped-care plan, and prescribe treatments that allow children and their parents or carers to follow this plan.

Treatment for flares of atopic eczema in children should be started as soon as signs and symptoms appear and continued for approximately 48 hours after symptoms subside.

CASE 14 Migraine

INFORMATION FOR THE DOCTOR

Name	Eddo Mpofo
Age	22
Social and family history	Single, no children, studying engineering at university
Past medical history	• Soft tissue R knee injury 6 months ago – had physiotherapy • Closed fracture L little finger 5 years ago • Migraine for 6 years • Greenstick fracture R radius 12 years ago • Asthma (mild) – triggered by cats and URTIs
Current medication	• Sumatriptan 100mg tablets; if symptoms recur, repeat dose after at least 2 hours. Maximum 300mg in 24h • Salbutamol inhaler PRN
Clinical values BMI BP	 23 122/76

INFORMATION FOR THE PATIENT

You are Eddo Mpofo, a 22-year-old university engineering student, who has come to discuss medication for your migraine. You have had migraine for six years. You get a one-sided, intensely painful headache (*"like someone sticking a knife through my upper teeth into my eye socket"*). The pain comes on without warning though sometimes you get a vague feeling that you will soon get a migraine. When this occurs, you need to take your sumatriptan tablets immediately.

When the headaches first started, you were told to take ibuprofen and paracetamol but this often failed to give relief so the GP you saw when you were at school prescribed sumatriptan, which worked well, until now, your last year at uni. The attacks have become frequent, almost weekly, are severe (8–9/10 without medication; 4/10 with medication) and can last anything between 3 and 12 hours. Now, when you get a migraine, you need to sleep and find it difficult to continue working with the headache, despite taking the sumatriptan. If you persist studying or working (as a part-time barman), you get nausea and vomiting and eventually have to lie down in a dark and quiet room. The migraine can occur at any time. If you haven't eaten, or if you are slightly dehydrated and working hard, you are more likely to have an attack. It has become difficult to attend lectures and to study.

During your A levels you tried amitriptyline but it gave you a dry mouth and an increased appetite. You put on 4kg in a month. The amitriptyline made you drowsy; studying and paying attention in class was difficult. Your GP took you off amitriptyline and told you to carry the sumatriptan tablets in your wallet and take them immediately. This worked until now. While the sumatriptan takes the edge off the pain, the nausea and vomiting seem to have worsened. You are not sure how much of the sumatriptan you are vomiting up. You have an important examination in six weeks. You would like new tablets that are more effective but something that does not make you feel tired and drowsy. Your opening statement on presentation today is *"I've come to discuss my migraine tablets"*.

Information to reveal if asked

General information about yourself:

- You are working hard at university and if you remain on track, it looks like you may be taken on by a large engineering company at which you did interesting work experience.
- You work as a barman a few nights a week.
- You play squash and do weights. You like to keep healthy.
- You live in a student house with 5 friends, including your girlfriend who is reading English Literature.
- You do not smoke or take illicit drugs.

Further details about your condition:

- Your migraine, you feel, is currently aggravated by exam stress. When you work hard, with intense concentration, to tight deadlines, reduce your sleep and skip meals, you are more likely to get migraine. As a result, you have learnt to be disciplined, especially in the two months leading up to exams, when you go to bed at specific times and get at least 6 hours of rest.

- If specifically asked about your lifestyle, you are a non-smoker. You drink 3 or 4 cans of beer with friends 2 – 3 nights per week. You share one or two bottles of wine with your girlfriend most weekends. You rarely get drunk.

- You do not think that any specific food or alcohol or activities trigger your migraine.

Your ideas:

- You think that the extra work and worry relating to your impending exams aggravated your migraine but you fear there is little you can do at present to reduce the stress.

- Your mum advised you to eat ginger to 'settle the stomach' but the smell of ginger aggravates your nausea. She also told you about feverfew but you think tablets are better than these folklore remedies.

- You really didn't get on with amitriptyline and you are reluctant to try it again because of your experience of its side-effects, particularly drowsiness and a 'woolly head'.

- You would prefer a tablet like sumatriptan, only stronger. You would prefer to avoid a daily tablet like amitriptyline.

Your concerns:

- You are worried about taking daily tablets in case you develop side-effects.

- You are worried about the effect the migraine is having on your work (studying and being attentive in lectures) and the effect on your social life. You are spending so much time sleeping off the pain, you hardly have any time left over to spend with your girlfriend.

Your expectations:

- You expect to get better medication for your migraine, preferably a tablet that you take only when you get the headache rather than preventative medication.

Medical history

You have mild asthma, worse with a cold. You only use your salbutamol inhaler when you have a cold or you are in contact with cats.

Social history

You are enjoying your time at university and happy with your favourable job interview.

Information to reveal if examined

An examination is not required.

SUGGESTED APPROACH TO THE CONSULTATION

Targeted history taking:

- What are Eddo's symptoms now? Describe the migraine. Where is the pain? Elicit intensity, duration, aggravating and relieving factors.

- Are there any new features (e.g. neurological deficit) to his migraine? Has he noticed any changes to his ability to think (cognition), any fever (recent travel/ HIV), headache in relation to exercise?

- Describe the nausea and vomiting. Does this occur without headache?

- What tablets does he use for treatment of the acute attacks? In terms of reducing pain (using a pain score), how effective is paracetamol, ibuprofen, sumatriptan, combination of sumatriptan with ibuprofen?

- What is the frequency and length of the attacks with and without medication?

- What activities does the migraine limit?

- For how long did he take amitriptyline, and at what dose? What were the side-effects?

- Did the side-effects interfere with his work and home life? How?

- Is he aware of other treatments (immediate and prophylactic)?

- Does he have any ideas about how he could reduce the intensity, duration, frequency and impact of his migraine?

- What are his concerns? Is he worried about the knock-on effect of disabling migraine on his studying, work and social life? Is he worried about headache being a symptom of a different illness?

- What are his expectations: did he have any specific medication in mind; did he want to discuss feverfew, did he want a neurology referral?

- What is his general health like? – get more information about his asthma.

Targeted examination:

- This case does not require the candidate to perform a targeted physical examination.

Clinical management:

- Empathise with Eddo: the migraines are severe, are adversely affecting his life, and are important to treat.

- He has been using his acute treatment as soon as gets the migraine, but he could try an anti-inflammatory (ibuprofen 400mg) or aspirin 900mg or paracetamol 1g with sumatriptan 100mg **and** an anti-emetic (such as prochlorperazine – oral or buccal). The alternative is to step up to zolmitriptan orodispersible – 2.5mg, repeated after not less than 2 hours, increasing to 5mg for subsequent attacks if 2.5mg is unsatisfactory. The maximum dose is 10mg in 24 hours. The step after orodispersible tablets is to use a nasal spray such as zolmitriptan nasal spray 5mg per spray (maximum dose 10mg in 24 hours). The step after that is to use sumatriptan 6mg subcutaneous injections. It may be useful to discuss the ladder for stepping up triptans (tablets to orodispersible/ wafers to nasal spray to injection) with Eddo.

- Discuss the option of prophylaxis: beta-blockers (propranolol) or topiramate are first-line choices, but in view of his asthma, beta-blockers are contra-indicated. Second-line options include a course of acupuncture or gabapentin (up to 1.2g/d, unlicensed indication).

- Establish the aims of treatment: to reduce the frequency, intensity, duration and impact of the attacks. However, the best that may be achieved with prophylaxis is a 50% reduction in frequency (and sometimes also a reduction in intensity) of the attacks.

- Address the patient's ideas: that exam stress may be intensifying his nausea and because he is vomiting up his sumatriptan, an alternative to a tablet may be needed. Orodispersible wafers are a good alternative; then nasal spray, then subcutaneous injections. Alternatively, he could try buccal prochlorperazine.

- Address the patient's concerns: that migraine prophylaxis medication is limited to amitriptyline, which for him has unacceptable side-effects. He may be interested in topiramate, acupuncture or riboflavin.

- Address his expectations: to get a prescription for different migraine tablets. Prescribe an evidence-based treatment, in line with *BNF* advice.

- Confirm his understanding of acute and prophylactic treatments for migraine.

- Safety-net: describe when and why Eddo should next consult.

Interpersonal skills:

This case tests the doctor's ability to present the treatment options (based on current UK guidance) to the patient. The options need to be communicated clearly, in a balanced manner and in jargon-free language so that the patient understands the potential benefits and risks. By the end of the discussion, the patient should feel sufficiently informed that he can make his own decision about which option is best for him.

Good communication with the patient:

- explores and empathises with the adverse impact of the migraines, and amitriptyline, on the patient's life.

- identifies key clinical clues, such as asthma being a contra-indication to the prescription of beta-blockers.

- responds to the patient's preferences for acute migraine medication, acknowledging the stress of impending exams.

- discusses medication options and encourages concordance – works in partnership with the patient.
- provides explanations that are relevant and understandable to the patient.

Poor communication with the patient:

- does not inform the patient of his options, both acute and prophylactic. The doctor prescribes an alternative medication without involving the patient in the decision.
- instructs the patient. The second half of the consultation is dominated by the doctor 'telling' the patient what to do, instead of a two-way conversation where the patient is asked about what he already knows and the important blanks filled in by the doctor in a conversational style.
- uses inappropriate or technical language.

BACKGROUND KNOWLEDGE REQUIRED FOR THIS CASE

NICE (CG150) (2012) **Headaches: Diagnosis and management of headaches in young people and adults.**

Acute treatment

1. Offer combination therapy with an **oral triptan and an NSAID**, or an oral triptan and **paracetamol**, for the acute treatment of migraine.
2. When prescribing a triptan start with the one that has the lowest acquisition cost; if this is consistently ineffective, try one or more alternative triptans.
3. Consider an **anti-emetic** in addition to other acute treatment for migraine even in the absence of nausea and vomiting.
4. Do not offer ergots or opioids for the acute treatment of migraine.
5. For people in whom oral preparations for the acute treatment of migraine are ineffective or not tolerated: offer a non-oral preparation of metoclopramide or prochlorperazine **and** consider adding a *non-oral NSAID or triptan* if these have not been tried.

Prophylactic treatment

1. Offer **topiramate** or **propranolol** for the prophylactic treatment of migraine according to the person's preference, comorbidities and risk of adverse events. Advise women and girls of childbearing potential that topiramate is associated with a risk of fetal malformations and can impair the effectiveness of hormonal contraceptives. Ensure they are offered suitable contraception.
2. If both topiramate and propranolol are unsuitable or ineffective, consider a course of up to 10 sessions of **acupuncture** over 5–8 weeks or **gabapentin**

(up to 1200mg per day) according to the person's preference, comorbidities and risk of adverse events.

3. For people who are already having treatment with another form of prophylaxis such as **amitriptyline**, and whose migraine is well controlled, continue the current treatment as required.

4. Advise those with migraine that **riboflavin** (400mg once a day) may be effective in reducing migraine frequency and intensity for some people.

Relevant literature

For diagnostic criteria and management guidelines, see www.bash.org.uk/

CASE 15 Nocturnal enuresis

INFORMATION FOR THE DOCTOR

Mrs Davina Jeffrey consults about her son Thomas's medical problem. Thomas is not present at the consultation.

Name	Thomas Jeffrey
Age	6
Social and family history	older of two children
Past medical history	• Pulled elbow 2 years ago • Otitis media 3 years ago
Current medication	None
Up to date with vaccinations Routine developmental checks – no problems noted	

INFORMATION FOR THE PATIENT

You are Mrs Davina Jeffrey, a 29-year-old woman who presents (without your 6-year-old son, Thomas) for advice on his bedwetting. You are concerned that Thomas still wets the bed at least 2 times per week. He has never been dry at night. He is dry during the day.

Thomas is a lovely child who is achieving well at school. He has lots of friends. However, you have declined the sleepovers to which Thomas has been invited. You think it would be embarrassing for him if he bed wets on a sleepover. You worry about him being teased.

Nobody in the family has had a bedwetting problem. You tried restricting Thomas's drinks at night but this has not made much difference.

You thought the problem would resolve by age 5. Thomas is six. You present to the doctor today with a few questions:

- Does Thomas have a problem predisposing him to bedwetting?
- Should he be investigated?
- Does he need tablet treatments? Is there anything else you should do?

Information to reveal if asked

General information about yourself:

- You are married to Adrian, a car mechanic. You are a part-time hairdresser. Your daughter Daisy is three and potty training is going well.
- Now that your daughter is 3, you would like to leave your children with your mum for a week so that you and your husband can go on holiday. The frequent changing and washing of bedding creates a burden of housework and you feel guilty approaching your 56-year-old mother.
- You sometimes feel irritated and frustrated with the amount of washing you have to do but neither you nor your husband get cross or angry with Thomas. You feel shouting at him will make him self-conscious and damage his self-confidence. You also don't want Daisy, who sleeps in a different room, picking up on the problem, or teasing her brother.

Further details about Thomas's condition:

- He has no medical problems and does not suffer from constipation or urine infections.
- The bed wetting occurs 2–4 times per week. Usually Thomas's bed is wet by the time you check at 11pm, but sometimes you only notice in the morning. It tends to be a large amount of urine. Thomas sleeps through the whole thing.

- Thomas seems fine during the day. He has not complained of pain on urination and he does not seem to go more often.

- You don't think Thomas drinks too much. He often has to be reminded to drink fluids and squash as he is a busy, active child and forgetful of fluids.

- All 3 bedrooms are upstairs. Your room is closest to the toilet, then Daisy's and then Thomas's. You leave a plugged-in night lamp to illuminate the corridor. You keep the corridor clear so Thomas can get to the toilet easily at night.

Your ideas:

- You think that the bedwetting should have stopped by age 5.

- You think Thomas has a 'weak' bladder.

- You have heard about alarms for bladder training but you are not sure about this. Daisy is a light sleeper and you are worried that she will be disturbed. Your husband needs to be alert to his work as a mechanic. You don't want him making mistakes and getting hurt at work because an interrupted night's sleep impairs his concentration.

Your concerns:

- You are worried about the social restrictions Thomas's bedwetting is having on him (no sleepovers or overnight trips) and the family (you can't leave him with your mum for some time away).

- You are concerned about how the family will respond to the idea of an alarm. Do you have to buy one? How effective is it?

Your expectations:

- You expect to get some information about bedwetting treatments and perhaps a prescription for some tablets.

Medical history

Thomas is healthy and you have no concerns about his development.

Social history

There are no family stresses, marital or financial issues at present.

Information to reveal if examined

An examination is not required.

SUGGESTED APPROACH TO THE CONSULTATION

Targeted history taking:

- Ask mum open questions to explore the nature of the bedwetting.

- Find out what has made her present today.

- Ask closed questions to identify potentially reversible contributory factors: constipation, urinary tract infections, diet, stress (school problems/family discord/moving house), diabetes mellitus, ease of access to a toilet or potty, night lights and bunk beds?

- Exclude red flags: neurological problems, behaviour problems, sleep apnoea.

- Elicit how the problem affects Thomas (embarrassment, social isolation, teasing by family members or friends).

- Elicit how the problem affects the family (parental anxiety/frustration/punishment/extra work of laundry/effect of interrupted sleep).

- Address her ideas that bedwetting should have ceased by age 6 by contextualising the problem: one in fifty 7-year-olds wets the bed more than once a week and 15% get better without treatment each year. There are different reasons for bedwetting: children who are passing large volumes at night may not be producing sufficient anti-diuretic hormone (ADH); small volumes may indicate small, irritable bladders; or the child may be sleeping so deeply that he is unaware of the sensation of a full bladder.

- Empathise with her concerns about the social restriction (sleepovers/ family holidays) but clarify whether these concerns are sufficient motivation for the family to want treatment. First-line treatment is with alarms. Though effective at achieving dryness in 2 out of 3 children at 3–6 months, alarms may be disruptive to the whole family. Second-line treatment in children 5 and over is with desmotabs or desmomelts (not nasal spray).

- Respond to mum's expectations for advice and a treatment plan by signposting to ERIC (enuresis resource and information centre: http://www.eric.org.uk/); discuss use of waterproof mattress coverings; avoid caffeine after 3pm; advise a fluid intake of 1–1.4L per day (recommended intake for a 6-year-old); encourage 4–7 toilet visits per day.

- Confirm Davina's understanding of primary nocturnal enuresis: its immediate treatment with sensible fluid intake/diet and regular toileting patterns; use of reward systems; and if these measures do not work, then alarms or desmotabs/desmomelts.

- Offer referral to the health visitor for ongoing treatment and support. Discuss that referral to secondary care in the absence of red flags is unlikely to add more to current management.

Interpersonal skills:

This case tests the doctor's ability to explore a problem with a concerned parent. The mother has not yet made up her mind about whether her child's problem needs treatment and seeks information about the issue from her GP. Once she has the information, she should be able to decide whether the problem is mild enough to adopt a wait and see policy, or severe enough to require treatment. The doctor is able to discuss step-wise treatment, including fluid/toilet advice, alarms and medication.

Good communication with the patient:

- listens attentively to the mother's concerns regarding the continued bedwetting and its impact on the family.
- displays empathy to the workload and financial burden the bedwetting creates.
- addresses the patient's specific expectations about a long-term solution and what could be done in the short term for sleepovers and holidays.
- sensitively explores the parents' frustration and obtains enough information to know if the child is being inappropriately punished or maltreated.
- phrases options in an open and unbiased manner; for example, the doctor could say *"I am reassured by what you have told me about Thomas's physical and social development. I think this problem will resolve in time as his hormones and bladder mature. There are a few things we could do to help Thomas. I'll talk through the options first and then perhaps I could give you a leaflet?"*

Poor communication with the patient:

- assumes that children under the age of 7 should not be treated and gives lifestyle advice only.
- does not explore child protection issues in a sensitive manner.
- fails to follow a step-wise approach to treatment, in line with current UK guidance.

BACKGROUND KNOWLEDGE REQUIRED FOR THIS CASE

NICE (Oct 2010), **Nocturnal enuresis: The management of bedwetting in children and young people**

- There are a number of different disturbances of physiology that may be associated with bedwetting. These disturbances may be categorised as sleep arousal difficulties, polyuria and bladder dysfunction. Bedwetting also often runs in families.
- Do not exclude younger children (for example, those under 7 years) from the management of bedwetting on the basis of age alone.

- Discuss with the parents or carers whether they need support.
- Consider whether or not it is appropriate to offer alarm or drug treatment.
- Address excessive or insufficient fluid intake or abnormal toileting patterns before starting other treatment for bedwetting in children and young people.
- Explain that reward systems with positive rewards for agreed behaviour rather than dry nights should be used either alone or in conjunction with other treatments for bedwetting. For example, rewards may be given for:
  - drinking recommended levels of fluid during the day
  - using the toilet to pass urine before sleep
  - engaging in management (for example, taking medication or helping to change sheets).
- Offer an alarm as the first-line treatment to children (age 5 and above) whose bedwetting has not responded to advice on fluids, toileting or an appropriate reward system, unless an alarm is considered undesirable or inappropriate (<1–2 wet beds per week) to the child or their parents.
- Assess the response to an alarm by 4 weeks but stop treatment if there are no early signs of response.
- Continue alarm treatment in responsive children until a minimum of 2 weeks' uninterrupted dry nights has been achieved.
- Inform patients that it may take a few weeks for the early signs of a response to the alarm to occur and that these may include:
  - smaller wet patches
  - waking to the alarm
  - the alarm going off later and fewer times per night
  - fewer wet nights.

Inform patients that dry nights may be a late sign of response to the alarm and may take weeks to achieve.

- Offer desmopressin to children and young people over the age of 5 years if:
  - rapid onset and/or short-term improvement in bedwetting is the priority of treatment or
  - an alarm is inappropriate or undesirable.
- Assess the response to desmopressin at 4 weeks and continue treatment for 3 months if there are signs of a response. Consider stopping if there are no signs of response.
- Refer children and young people with bedwetting that has not responded to courses of treatment with an alarm and/or desmopressin. Specialists could consider a prescription of desmopressin combined with an anti-cholinergic; or a prescription of imipramine.

CASE 16 Psoriasis

INFORMATION FOR THE DOCTOR

Susie Neilson consults about her daughter Anna's medical problem. Anna is not present at the consultation.

Name	Anna Neilson
Age	12
Social and family history	Daughter of Susie Neilson, divorced
Past medical history	• Guttate psoriasis 4 months ago • Sore throat – treated with penicillin × 10 days 4 months ago • Flat feet 4 years ago
Current medication	• Doublebase cream 500mg apply thrice daily • Eumovate once daily to affected areas • Oilatum bath emollient – use daily in bath

INFORMATION FOR THE PATIENT

You are Susie Neilson, 32-year-old mother of Anna, a 12-year-old who developed guttate psoriasis suddenly four months ago following a throat infection, which was treated with antibiotics. Thereafter, Anna was prescribed several different emollient creams for the psoriasis. At the moment, Anna bathes in baby-oil softened water using a moisturising soap. She towels dry and applies an emollient. A few minutes later, she applies Eumovate steroid cream. She applies the emollients at least twice daily, and although well tolerated, this regime is time-consuming. You worry about the long-term effect of steroids on the skin; *"it thins the skin".*

You saw an internet article and have printed out the advertisement to discuss with the doctor.

Al-Preve Miracle Cure

After bathing/showering with a glycerine soap, just peel a banana, and rub the inner soft skin (the one next to the banana) on your patch of psoriasis. The peel is the scrub. Rub it in thoroughly. Later, once your skin has absorbed the oils from the peel, we suggest you use a common gentle skin cream to help keep the psoriasis patch soft. Our best-selling cream is 'Al-Preve', which does not contain the dyes and perfumes that make the psoriasis sting. It is a simple cream with vitamins and is made from entirely natural ingredients. If you discontinue all other products and use 'Al-Preve' at least once a day, the nasty, white flaky skin will soften up and eventually you will see a miraculous thing – pink healthy skin emerging.

You have not spoken to Anna about the 'Miracle Cure' because you wanted to get the doctor's opinion first. The internet article says all other creams should be discontinued, presumably because they contain non-natural, synthetic ingredients. Does this include Anna's prescribed emollient? You think Anna will use the 'Miracle Cure', especially if it simplifies and shortens the daily routine. You are not sure how Anna would feel about the smell of bananas though. You expect Anna to use the cream for two or three months. Hopefully, this cream will push the guttate psoriasis into complete remission. A poor result would be the lack of a cure and the development of chronic psoriasis. You think that because the 'Miracle Cure' is made from natural ingredients, it should not cause any harm, unlike steroids. It costs £25 per tube, per month. You are not aware of other treatments such as phototherapy, which are available on the NHS.

Anna is getting self-conscious about her appearance. She now refuses to swim; chlorine also stings. Anna does not want to wear summer clothes despite the heat, because people might see the plaques. Also, the whole routine takes so long. Anna has been late for school on a few occasions. You want to know what is the best course of action for Anna. You don't mind paying for the 'Miracle Cure' if you think it will help Anna.

You present to the doctor expecting to discuss 'Al-Preve' cream for Anna's psoriasis.

Information to reveal if asked

General information about yourself and Anna:

- You had acne as a teenager, which left you feeling shy and under-confident. You want Anna to have good skin and not be self-conscious.

- Anna is a quiet and happy girl. She has a group of friends who are interested in music. Anna plays piano.

- Anna seems happy at school and as far as you know, does not have a boyfriend, although she quite likes Nick, who also attends her school.

Further details about Anna's condition:

- Anna developed guttate psoriasis very quickly after a bad Strep sore throat.

- If specifically asked, she had and still has lots of small red separate spots ('like coins') on her front, back, tops of thighs and arms. They feel raised but are not particularly thick. They were very itchy, worse in hot weather or hot showers, but less itchy now. Anna still scratches and the itch seems to get worse when she is stressed. You found Anna 'itched a lot' during a music exam.

Your ideas:

- You and Anna thought the guttate psoriasis would be self-limiting and are surprised that it persisted this long. You expected the prescription creams to make the plaques vanish. The plaques are still present and are itchy and unsightly. You think that Anna is good about applying her creams, but they are not sufficiently effective.

- You think the doctor may want to give a stronger steroid cream and you worry about this thinning and ageing Anna's skin.

- If the doctor offers to prescribe a stronger steroid or a different skin cream, you are a bit hesitant (*"Do they contain natural ingredients?"*) and want to know about possible side-effects. You want to know what the doctor thinks of the 'Al-Preve' cream.

Your concerns:

- You are worried about Anna becoming self-conscious.

- You hope this has not turned into a long-term skin problem.

Your expectations:

- You expect to get an opinion on 'Al-Preve' Cream and advice on how to help Anna get better.

Medical history

Anna is usually fit and healthy.

Social history

You are divorced. Anna gets on well with her dad, whom she sees regularly. Nobody in your family has psoriasis and your ex-husband thinks his uncle may have had psoriasis.

Information to reveal if examined

Examination is not necessary.

SUGGESTED APPROACH TO THE CONSULTATION

Targeted history taking:

- What type of psoriasis does Anna have? Where are the lesions and how much of her skin is affected? Would mum grade Anna's skin as clear, nearly clear, mild, moderate, severe or very severe? Why?

- How is the psoriasis affecting Anna? What is the impact of psoriasis on school and home life? How is she coping with her psoriasis and her treatments? Is she distressed by having the skin lesions? What is Anna's mood like?

- What is her current treatment regime? What is good and what is bad with the current treatments?

- What does Anna think of the 'Miracle Cure'? Is she likely to use the treatment regime as directed?

- What expectations do Anna and/or Susie have of the cream? What would be a good result?

- What could the possible harms be of using this cream? How expensive is it?

- What does Susie think about the other evidence-based treatments, available on the NHS, for Anna?

- What are Susie's expectations of this consultation: your opinion on the product, your advice regarding the treatment of psoriasis, a change in Anna's prescriptions, or a referral to dermatology?

Targeted examination:

- This case does not require the candidate to perform a targeted physical examination.

Clinical management:

- Address the mother's ideas: that guttate psoriasis is self-limiting. Discuss the natural history of guttate psoriasis – it often runs a self-limited course, lasting from a few weeks to a few months, but in approximately two-thirds of cases, it develops into chronic plaque-type psoriasis. Be sensitive and empathetic. Be hopeful – it may be too early to assume that it has become a chronic disease.

- Address the mother's concerns: that steroid creams thin and damage the skin. Discuss the role of steroid. Comment on the strength of steroid cream previously prescribed and how this deviates from current guidance where a more potent corticosteroid (such as Betnovate) applied once daily or calcipotriol (e.g. Dovonex) applied once daily is advised.

- Address the mother's expectations: of inducing remission. Anna needs to be re-examined – is the guttate psoriasis taking a bit longer than expected to clear (probably because it has been treated with too low a potency steroid), or has it developed into chronic type psoriasis? Discuss the availability of treatment options such as vitamin D analogues (e.g. Dovonex), phototherapy or a coal-tar preparation, such as Exorex, which contains extracts from bananas. All these treatments are available on the NHS.

- Discuss the likelihood of 'Al-Preve' inducing remission, being used regularly, and its possible harms. Give your opinion of the internet regime, its possible benefits and harms. Once the information is provided, allow Susie to evaluate the risks and benefits of the treatment. Negotiate and develop a shared plan.

- Incorporate Anna's and Susie's values and preferences for treatment. If Susie wants to use 'Al-Preve', then negotiate a trial of treatment. How would Susie decide whether the cream is beneficial? Arrange follow-up against agreed success criteria.

- Discuss the availability of support from other team members, such as the practice nurse who has an interest in dermatology.

- If required, provide written information in support of the discussion.

Interpersonal skills:

This case tests several important skills, namely, the doctor's ability to:

- assess the physical and psychological impact of a dermatological condition on the patient and her family, that is, to undertake a *holistic* assessment

- negotiate a management plan

- prescribe appropriately in children/young adults, in line with current UK guidance.

Good communication with the patient:

- explores and acknowledges the reasons for the mother's attendance – her wish to do more for her daughter; concerns about Anna's recent self-conscious behaviour; and her fear that long-term use of steroid cream may be harmful to Anna's skin.

- appreciates that Susie may have an underlying fear that her daughter's guttate psoriasis may be evolving into a chronic plaque-type disease.

- explores her expectations of treatment. By discussing the natural history of the disease and explaining how treatments work, Susie is empowered.

- achieves a shared understanding, and negotiates an appropriate and acceptable management plan.

- therefore, finalising on a decision for which both parties take responsibility, maintains the doctor–patient relationship.

Poor communication with the patient:

- fails to appreciate that bringing in an article on a 'Miracle Cure' may be Susie's attempt at signalling concerns with Anna's current treatment.

- dismisses the 'Miracle Cure' out of hand without taking time to consider with Susie its possible acceptability, benefits and drawbacks.

- is patronising and fails to foster a therapeutic doctor–patient relationship.

BACKGROUND KNOWLEDGE REQUIRED FOR THIS CASE

NICE CG153 (2012) **Psoriasis: The assessment and management of psoriasis**

For people with any type of psoriasis assess:

- disease severity
- the impact of disease on physical, psychological and social wellbeing
- whether they have psoriatic arthritis
- the presence of comorbidities.

When assessing the disease severity in any healthcare setting, record:

- a classification of clear, nearly clear, mild, moderate, severe or very severe
- the body surface area affected – is 10% or more of the skin surface area covered by plaque?
- any involvement of nails, high-impact and difficult-to-treat sites (for example, the face, scalp, palms, soles, flexures and genitals)
- any systemic upset such as fever and malaise, which are common in unstable forms of psoriasis such as erythroderma or generalised pustular psoriasis.

Assess the impact of any type of psoriasis on physical, psychological and social wellbeing by asking:

- what aspects of their daily living are affected by the person's psoriasis
- how the person is coping with their skin condition and any treatments they are using
- if they need further advice or support
- if their psoriasis has an impact on their mood
- if their psoriasis causes them distress (be aware the patient may have levels of distress and not be clinically depressed)
- if their condition has any impact on their family or carers.

Treatment

First-line therapy describes traditional topical therapies (such as corticosteroids, vitamin D and vitamin D analogues, dithranol and tar preparations).

Second-line therapy includes the phototherapies (broad- or narrow-band ultraviolet B light and psoralen plus UVA light [PUVA]) and systemic non-biological agents such as ciclosporin, methotrexate and acitretin.

Third-line therapy refers to systemic biological therapies such as the tumour necrosis factor antagonists adalimumab, etanercept and infliximab, and the monoclonal antibody ustekinumab that targets interleukin-12 (IL-12) and IL-23.

'Children' refers to those up to 12 years, who become 'young people' thereafter, before merging with the adult population by 18 years of age.

Topical treatment of psoriasis affecting the trunk and limbs

Children

- For children and young people with trunk or limb psoriasis consider either calcipotriol (e.g. Dovonex) applied once daily (only for those over 6 years of age) or a potent corticosteroid (e.g. Betnovate) applied once daily (only for those over 1 year of age).

Adults

- Offer a potent corticosteroid (e.g. Betnovate) applied once daily plus vitamin D or a vitamin D analogue (e.g. Dovonex) applied once daily (applied separately, one in the morning and the other in the evening) for up to 4 weeks as initial treatment for adults with trunk or limb psoriasis.
- If once-daily application of a potent corticosteroid plus once-daily application of vitamin D (e.g. Dovobet) or a vitamin D analogue (e.g. Dovonex) does not result in clearance, near clearance or satisfactory control of trunk or limb psoriasis in adults after a maximum of 8 weeks, offer vitamin D or a vitamin D analogue alone (e.g. Dovonex) applied twice daily.
- If twice-daily application of vitamin D or a vitamin D analogue (e.g. Dovonex) does not result in clearance, near clearance or satisfactory control of trunk or limb psoriasis in adults after 8–12 weeks, offer either:
  ○ a potent corticosteroid (e.g. Dermovate) applied twice daily for up to 4 weeks
  or
  ○ a coal tar preparation (e.g. Exorex) applied once or twice daily.
- If a twice-daily potent corticosteroid or coal tar preparation cannot be used or a once-daily preparation would improve adherence in adults, offer a combined product containing calcipotriol monohydrate and betamethasone dipropionate (e.g. Taclonex) applied once daily for up to 4 weeks.
- Offer treatment with very potent corticosteroids in adults with trunk or limb psoriasis only in specialist settings under careful supervision when other topical treatment strategies have failed for a maximum period of 4 weeks.
- Consider short-contact dithranol for treatment-resistant psoriasis of the trunk or limbs and either give educational support for self-use **or** ensure treatment is given in a specialist setting.

CASE 17 Tonsillitis

INFORMATION FOR THE DOCTOR

Name	Pippa Whittaker
Age	37
Social and family history	Married, with 3 children
Past medical history	• R patello-femoral maltracking 7 years ago – had physiotherapy • Traumatic fractured right ankle 8 years ago • L shoulder pain 10 years ago – posture related
Current medication	Marvelon CHC take 1 tablet daily for 21 days, then have a 7 day break
Clinical values BP Height Weight BMI	*last seen 3 months ago* 124/78 172cm 74kg 25

INFORMATION FOR THE PATIENT

You are Pippa Whittaker, a 37-year-old senior administrator at a financial services company. You started to feel unwell four days ago. You have been experiencing hot and cold temperature spells and feel very tired. When you feel cold, you shiver and cannot get warm. You have a generalised dull headache and a very sore throat with difficulty eating. You are so tired, you fell asleep at 8pm last night and slept right through to the morning. This is very unlike you. You felt too ill and tired to drive to work today. You plan to work from home today.

The illness started four days ago, at the same time as your daughter's illness. Your 3-year-old girl is at nursery and seems to have caught something that is going around nursery.

You do not have a history of recurrent sore throats. You just want to get 'checked out' and for the doctor to confirm you have a self-limiting viral illness.

You present to the doctor wishing to discuss your flu-like symptoms. Your opening statement is *"I feel so washed out, I think I may actually have man-flu"*.

Information to reveal if asked

General information about yourself:

- You work at a financial services company in a well-paid and demanding job.
- Work is challenging but rewarding. However, to have a career like yours and three children requires concentration and organisation. Your husband, an IT consultant, and your au pair help at home.

Further details about your condition:

- If specifically asked, you do not have cough, urinary symptoms, or diarrhoea and vomiting. You have a sore throat and think your neck glands are swollen. It hurts to swallow but it is not too painful (4/10).
- You are sleeping too long, but you have not had feverish dreams or delirium.
- You tried taking regular paracetamol for the fever, which has helped. You took paracetamol an hour before this consultation.
- You are very rarely ill. You do not have any long-term illnesses, nor do you take any medication that may be lowering your immunity.

Your ideas:

- You think that you have the same viral illness as your daughter and just need some time at home to recover.

Your concerns:

- You are worried that if you didn't consult the doctor for an examination, you are in danger of ignoring a serious illness.

- Your sister-in-law had bacterial endocarditis last year which presented as a feverish illness, which she ignored until she became very ill. Now your sister-in-law has a damaged heart valve.

Your expectations:

- You just want to get 'checked out' and for the doctor to confirm you have a self-limiting viral illness.

- You expect to be examined and reassured. You do not want antibiotics; you prefer homeopathic medicines.

Medical history

You are in good general health, and currently using Marvelon for contraception.

Social history

You are happily married with a busy and full social life.

Information to reveal if examined

- If the doctor asks to examine your tonsils, hand him/her a picture of enlarged, follicular tonsils:

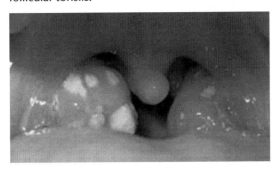

Reproduced from: http://mbahdukunbagong.blogspot.co.uk/2011/05/tonsilitis.html

- If the doctor assesses for cervical lymphadenopathy, hand a card reading *"Cervical lymphadenopathy is present"*.

- If the doctor measures your temperature, hand a card – temperature recorded as 37.8°C.

SUGGESTED APPROACH TO THE CONSULTATION

Targeted history taking:

- What are her current symptoms?

- For how long has she had these symptoms?

- Does she have cough, sore throat, earache, urinary symptoms, or diarrhoea and vomiting?

- In what way are the symptoms affecting her home and work life?

- Does the fever disturb sleep?

- What treatments has she tried already?

- Does she have any illnesses or does she take any medication that may be lowering her immunity?

- What does she think is causing her illness?

- Does she have a past history of recurrent infection, or complicated illness? Does she have any particular concerns?

- What are her expectations of this consultation: an examination and reassurance, further investigation, medication, a sick note?

- What is her general health like – is she still taking contraception?

Targeted examination:

- A targeted examination of the temperature, throat and neck is required.

Clinical management:

- Discuss the difficulty in diagnosing viral versus bacterial tonsillitis. The follicular appearance, the history of fever and malaise point to a bacterial infection.

- Explain that swabs are not routinely indicated in patients whose immunity is not compromised.

- Discuss the Centor criteria, a validated system for grading the severity of sore throats. As Pippa has pus, the absence of a cough, tender cervical lymph nodes and a history of fever, she has a severe infection according to the Centor criteria. Her chances of having a bacterial Group A beta-haemolytic streptococcal infection are in the region of 25–86%. Hence, antibiotics could be prescribed, either today or by issuing a delayed script. However, if she did not take antibiotics, her chances of being symptom-free by day 7 are high (85% of patients with sore throat, regardless of the causative organism, are symptom-free by day 7).

- Address the patient's ideas: she believes she has a self-limiting viral infection. In the absence of near-patient testing, you are unable to confirm or disprove this belief. Whether this is viral or bacterial sore throat, the most effective treatment is analgesia. Ibuprofen 400mg TDS or paracetamol 1g QDS may be all that is required.

- Address the patient's concerns: ignoring an illness in its early stages can result in potentially serious complications. Antibiotics for streptococcal sore throat can reduce the incidence of acute rheumatic fever and glomerulonephritis, both of which are rare in the UK. SIGN (2010) does not advise antibiotic prescription simply to prevent rheumatic fever or glomerular nephritis.

- Address the patient's expectations: she prefers homeopathic remedies and would prefer not to take antibiotics. SIGN guidance (2010): "Echinacea purpurea is not recommended for the treatment of sore throat". However, you could discuss the use of a delayed script, especially if symptoms worsen despite regular ibuprofen use. Safety-net – discuss the symptoms of the best-case and worst-case scenarios and outline what she should do in their eventuality.

- If you do prescribe, consider antipyretic analgesics and/or antibiotics – SIGN guidelines (2010) recommend penicillin V 500mg four times daily for 10 days in severe cases. If penicillin V is used, a 10-day course should be prescribed. Alternatively, erythromycin or azithromycin can be used as a 5-day course.

- If antibiotics are used, no extra precautions with contraceptives are required, unless she develops diarrhoea or vomiting, which may interfere with Pill absorption.

Interpersonal skills:

Good communication with the patient:

- responds to the person's concerns with understanding – discusses the rare complications of bacterial tonsillitis in a sensitive and understandable manner.

- backs his or her own judgement appropriately – discusses the Centor criteria, discusses effective treatments and the pros and cons of each treatment, leaving the final choice to the patient.

- acts in an open and non-judgemental manner – respects the patient's decision not to have antibiotics but allows for re-consultation or provides a delayed script should symptoms worsen.

Poor communication with the patient:

- does not work through the diagnostic sieve to elicit why the patient feels 'unwell and feverish'.

- does not inquire sufficiently about the patient's perspective and health understanding – her niggling concern about serious complications from a seemingly self-limiting illness.

- uses a rigid approach to consulting that is insufficiently responsive to the patient's contribution – launches into a discussion about antibiotics without appreciating the patient's preference for homeopathic medicines.

- fails to empower the patient – fails to safety-net.

BACKGROUND KNOWLEDGE REQUIRED FOR THIS CASE

SIGN (2010) **Management of sore throat and indications for tonsillectomy**
http://www.sign.ac.uk/pdf/qrg117.pdf

The Centor score gives one point each for:

- tonsillar exudate
- tender anterior cervical lymph nodes
- history of fever
- absence of cough.

The likelihood of group A beta-haemolytic streptococcus (GABHS) infection increases with increasing score, and is 25–86% with a score of 4, and 2–23% with a score of 1, depending upon age, local prevalence and seasonal variation.

Streptococcal infection is most likely in the 5–15 year old age group and gets progressively less likely in younger or older patients. The score is not validated for use in children under three years of age.

If breathing difficulty is present, urgent referral to hospital is mandatory and attempts to examine the throat should be avoided.

Diagnosis of a sore throat does not mean that an antibiotic has to be administered. Adequate analgesia will usually be all that is required. Ibuprofen 400mg three times daily is recommended for relief of fever, headache and throat pain in adults.

Sore throat should not be treated with antibiotics specifically to prevent the development of possible complications, such as rheumatic fever and acute glomerulonephritis.

CASE 18 **Overdose**

INFORMATION FOR THE DOCTOR

Name	Fiona McMinn
Age	38
Social and family history	Married, one child
Past medical history	• Alcohol problem drinking • Low mood

The medical record of her **last consultation** in surgery two weeks ago reads:

"Cut down drinking to weekends and two days per week. No problems at work or with family. Citalopram helped and feeling better. Still getting a few low days. Plan: continue citalopram for a further four months. Review in six to eight weeks."

Current medication	Citalopram 20mg once daily
Blood tests Full blood count Liver function tests	*Blood tests done two years ago* normal normal
BP	134/84

Summary of the A&E letter from last week:

- *"Overdose of paracetamol and salicylates*
- *Alcohol involvement: suspected*
- *Psychoactive drug involvement: no/information not available*
- *Investigation: biochemistry, ECG, haematology*
- *Treatment: Parvolex and fluids*
- *Repeat bloods normal*
- *Assessed by psychiatry. Discharged – follow-up by GP"*

INFORMATION FOR THE PATIENT

You are Fiona McMinn, a 38-year-old care worker, who has come to see the GP for a sick note. You have self-certified for the last week of illness but feel unable to return to work as yet. The Mental Health nurse who assessed you in hospital last week also advised you to see the GP to get more tablets; they only supplied 7 days of citalopram 40mg tablets.

You took three overdoses last week. The admission to hospital occurred following the last overdose. The first overdose involved ten paracetamol; the second seven coproxamol and the third involved a combination of twenty citalopram and fifteen ibuprofen. You took the third overdose after you dropped off your child at school.

You took the tablets with vodka in the woods and sat there intending to die. Your husband, who does not routinely telephone you during the day, happened to call you on your mobile. When you told him you'd taken pills, he called for an ambulance and came to the woods to find you.

You are not sure how you feel about the suicide attempt now. You are glad you did not die. Since the overdose, you have been able to talk more openly with your husband. You have discussed the stresses in your life over the past year: your dad being ill with end-stage heart failure; the stress that working with the elderly causes; and coping with a child who has behavioural difficulties.

You present to the doctor expecting to get a sick note for work. You want to return to work in two weeks. The hospital psychiatrist increased the citalopram to 40mg once daily and said you'd feel better after 3 weeks on medication. Your opening statement is *"I need a prescription for more antidepressants please"*.

Information to reveal if asked

General information about yourself:

- You work for a care company, caring mainly for elderly patients. You provide a home-help service and go into their homes to see that they have taken their medication, got themselves out of bed and washed, etc.

- You do not enjoy this job. You started this work when you husband was made redundant 2 years ago. He now has a job, but you have debts, making this job necessary.

- You do not have many friends locally. A lot of people moved out of the area when the biggest employer, an engineering company, closed.

Further details about your condition:

- You have been sad for six months. You twice saw another doctor at the practice for help with your depression and alcohol problems. You were prescribed citalopram five weeks ago. When reviewed two weeks ago, things had seemed better but then you felt low again.
- You are adamant that you do not wish to join AA, having attended and disliked your first meeting.
- You do not feel hopeless about the future, just sad about the pain your father is in. You see elderly people at work and how lonely and helpless they are. You imagine your father living in his home more than 3 hours' drive away, dying slowly of an incurable illness.
- You do not think about harming yourself but you worry about how easy it felt for you to take the overdoses last week.
- Nothing precipitated last week's overdose. It was the accumulation of the ongoing stresses.

Your ideas:

- You feel that you lack control over events in your life and last week, you wanted your problems to go away. You are not sure that you really wanted to die; you now think you'd acted impulsively. You used tablets that were in the house at the time; you did not stockpile tablets or try to buy a large number of new tablets.
- You think you are depressed. You think about the pain of illness all the time. The people you look after are in pain. You dad is in pain. You feel tired and hopeless.

Your concerns:

- You are worried about how easy it was to sit in the woods, drink the vodka and take the tablets. It felt like such a release from the pain.
- When you drink, the pain goes away for a while and you feel warm and safe.
- You know that your husband will look after your daughter. She can be confrontational and violent towards you but is much calmer with your husband.

Your expectations:

- You expect to get a prescription for more tablets.
- You don't want to return to work. The hospital doctor said it might take three weeks for the tablets to work properly, so you hope the doctor will sign you off for a further two weeks.

Medical history

You are usually healthy. You enjoy having a drink but have not had medical problems due to alcohol or alcohol-related accidents or trouble with employers or police because of alcohol.

Social history

You are married and have a 6-year-old child, Abi. Your relationship with Abi is difficult. Abi can be rude and boisterous, and is prone to tantrums. Other mothers think you cannot discipline your daughter and dislike you. You feel unsupported by your husband who has an easier relationship with Abi.

Information to reveal if examined

- With last week's suicide attempt, you hadn't written a note or willed gifts to people.

- You are not sure why you answered your phone when your husband called. You did not contact him and you had chosen an isolated place in the woods where your attempt was unlikely to be interrupted.

- You didn't think suicide would solve your problems. You just wanted to sleep; to get some rest from your feelings.

- You didn't think that a box of citalopram and a handful of ibuprofen washed down with vodka would kill you. You assumed that no lasting damage could be done to your body by what you'd taken, especially if your stomach was pumped. You had consumed half a bottle of vodka before taking the pills.

- You are not sure if you wanted to or still want to die. Sometimes it would feel like a relief. Sometimes you think you could be inflicting pain on your family.

- You now feel foolish. You feel tired. You also feel that your husband now understands the stress of your job and the stress of looking after your daughter. You hope that he will be more supportive.

SUGGESTED APPROACH TO THE CONSULTATION

Targeted history taking:

- Ask for further information regarding the circumstances of the overdose.
- Particularly, ask whether she was alone when she overdosed; did she time it such that she was unlikely to be found; whether she took precautions against being rescued; if she called anybody after taking the overdose; whether she wrote a suicide note or made any final plans?
- Was this an impulsive or premeditated act?
- How does she feel about the overdose now?
- Also enquire as to her feelings before the overdose – was she sad for most of the time?
- Does she feel hopeless about the future?
- Was this the first time she has tried to harm herself?
- Does she still think about harming herself?
- Were there any events that precipitated the act?
- What are her social circumstances: who lives with her at home and what job does she do?
- What advice did the hospital give? Has follow-up been arranged?
- What are her expectations of this consultation: a sick note, referral to the practice counsellor or psychiatry or alcohol services, discussion on recent overdose?
- Are there any ongoing general health problems that need to be managed? In particular, explore the role that alcohol played in the overdose and her relationship to alcohol at present.

Targeted examination:

- A mental state examination and assessment of suicide risk is required.

Clinical management:

- It is important to form a good relationship with the patient. A trusting and comfortable relationship is required for disclosure of her history and feelings.
- Assess her suicide risk. While there are scales available for assessing suicide risk, such as Pierce's Suicidal Intention Scale and Beck's Suicidal Intention Scale, it is most important to rule out red flags (see *Background medical knowledge required for this case*).
- Assess her support networks and co-create a safety plan.
- Address the patient's ideas: that she lacks control over the current events in her life and the feelings she has. Consider asking her what she could do to

resist suicidal thoughts and actions to take if the thoughts became stronger or persistent. Focus on the immediate safety issues, such as getting through this day and this week.

- Address the patient's concerns: that she found it so easy to act on a fleeting impulse. Ask her what else she could do to prevent these impulses – she may identify that if she were not under the influence of alcohol, she would be less impulsive. Ask her what else she could do if these impulses recurred; who could she phone? Does she have the telephone numbers of professional, voluntary and out of hours support readily available?

- Address the patient's expectations: for a sick note and a script for citalopram. It may be useful to ask the patient if time away from work increases her social isolation, or whether the return to work would expose her to further stress. With regard to medication, usually a script for a one-week supply is given. This could be tied in with supportive follow-up and could be phrased as *"I want to support you and you need you to know that we are here for you until you feel better.... Can I see you tomorrow/in the next couple of days/next week and see how you are getting on?"*

- Arrange follow-up either in surgery or by telephone. Usually patients at low risk of suicide need review in a week; high-risk patients with red flag signs require referral to the mental health team.

Interpersonal skills:

Good communication with the patient:

- acknowledges her despair, perceived losses and daily difficulties.
- helps her to deal with her sense of hopelessness and lack of control by providing empathetic support – the doctor helps her to establish new and accessible goals.
- focuses on working out daily problems rather than achieving psychological insight.
- negotiation regarding the sick note, request for further medication and follow-up is undertaken in a sensitive and considerate manner.

Poor communication with the patient:

- lacks empathy. The doctor is unable to develop rapport or forge a trusting relationship in which the patient feels she can voice her feelings or seek the support she wants.
- is unable to assess suicide risk properly. The open questions about her last attempt and her current feelings are not followed up by specific questions on suicide intent.
- fails to co-create a safety plan. The patient is not helped to explore her reasons for living and actions to take to challenge suicidal thoughts.

BACKGROUND KNOWLEDGE REQUIRED FOR THIS CASE

Cole-King, A *et al.* **Suicide Mitigation in Primary Care.**
http://www.connectingwithpeople.org/sites/default/files/
SuicideMitigationInPrimaryCareFactsheet_0612.pdf

All aspects of suicidal thoughts need to be identified:

- Perception of the future as persistently negative and hopeless;
- Nature of the suicidal thoughts, i.e. frequency, intensity, persistence, etc.;
- Degree of suicide intent:
    - planning and preparation for suicide attempt
    - putting affairs in order;
- Ability to resist acting *on* their thoughts of suicide or self-harm.

The following are **'red flag'** signs and indicate when a patient requires urgent specialist advice/input:

- Well-formed suicidal plans and preparations
- Recent worsening of distress
- Hopelessness: especially if only able to see a brief future, *"nothing to live for"*, guilt, *"I'm a burden"*
- Distressing psychotic phenomena, persecutory and nihilistic delusions; command hallucinations perceived as omnipotent
- Sense of 'entrapment'
- Pain/chronic medical illness
- Perception of lack of social support: no confidants
- Major relationship instability
- Recently bereaved.

If 'red flag' warning signs/immediate risk of suicidal behaviour (and especially if a patient is unknown to the GP) the patient will require:

- immediate discussion with/referral to mental health services
- a robust safety plan
- adequate support
- removal of access to means if possible.

How to co-create a safety plan:

The key is to enable the patient to generate their own reasons for living. A safety plan will usually include:

- actions or strategies to help resist suicidal thoughts
- names of supportive family and friends
- professional support
- voluntary support organisations

- agreed actions to take when suicidal thoughts become stronger and/or more persistent;
- access to out of hours support (when people may be at their most vulnerable and 'the system' is not obvious to distressed patients or their carers)
- use the 'Feeling on the Edge' resource: www.rcpsych.ac.uk/mentalhealthinfo/problems/feelingontheedge.aspx

Also see http://learning.bmj.com/learning/module-intro/suicide-prevention-primary-care.html?moduleId=10019936

CASE 19 Palpitations

INFORMATION FOR THE DOCTOR

Name	Neil Maskell
Age	41
Social and family history	Divorced
Past medical history	• Travel advice 9 years ago • Upper GI endoscopy 14 years ago
Current medication	None
Tests Urine dipstix BP Height Weight BMI	*Tests done five months ago (insurance medical)* no glucose, protein or blood detected 114/81 172cm 71kg 25

INFORMATION FOR THE PATIENT

You are Neil Maskell, a 41-year-old heating engineer, who has come to discuss the 'funny heartbeats' you have been experiencing over the last two days. The disturbing heartbeats started suddenly, while at work. You don't recall a particular activity, food, or event that triggered the 'funny beats'. You suddenly became aware of the forceful beating of your heart. By forceful you mean that when you placed your hand on your chest, you could feel the chest wall and breastbone pounding and moving. Your heart also seemed to miss a beat, have a forceful beat and then speed up for a minute or two. When you took your pulse during an episode, it was 80 but you were not sure if it was regular. The pounding beating was followed by a normal period, of at least one hour. Your heartbeat feels normal now.

The forceful heartbeats started two days ago and kept recurring, every few hours. The longest it lasted was ten minutes. You were aware of your heartbeat, intermittently throughout your night shift and when you tried to rest at home. You can't make it worse and you can't make it better. You have to walk up stairs at work and this does not provoke 'funny beats'. When these 'funny beats' occur, you do not have chest pain or shortness of breath. Your concentration is not impaired; you are not dizzy or light-headed.

You present to the doctor expecting an examination and some heart tests. Your opening statement is *"I'm a bit worried about my heart"*.

Information to reveal if asked

General information about yourself:

- You work in an engineering firm, but your job is mainly desk-based and administrative now.

- You went through a stressful divorce last year, but 'a new regime' has taken over this year. You now feel settled and happy in your new relationship.

- You don't use OTC medication, illicit drugs or take regular medication.

- If asked about caffeine, you say you are a tea drinker – you drink approximately six cups of strong tea each day.

Further details about your condition:

- The 'funny heartbeats' are not associated with chest pain, shortness of breath or light-headedness. You are not feeling generally stressed, anxious or depressed.

- You are well and have not lost weight or had health problems recently.

- If specifically asked about your lifestyle, you now smoke 10 cigarettes per day. Your girlfriend made you cut down this year. You previously smoked 20 per day for 20 years.

- You have also cut down alcohol from 4 beers a night to now only drinking a couple of cans on weekends.
- You last had your cholesterol measured 10 years ago and didn't have any problems. Your urine test for an insurance medical recently didn't pick up diabetes.
- Except for weekly golf, you do not get much exercise.

Your ideas:

- You think with your family history of cardiac disease, you cannot ignore these symptoms. When your dad died of an arrhythmia at age 64, your mum said he should have had a pacemaker.
- You think you may have 'heart damage'; these 'funny beats' are symptoms of damage. You think if the doctor did some tests, he or she would pick up exactly how much damage there is. If your heart circuits are damaged, perhaps you'll need a pacemaker.

Your concerns:

- You are worried about 'heart damage' because you have a family history of cardiac disease and 'genetically' may have a weak heart. Your dad died of an arrhythmia at age 64 and your older sister had an MI last year at age 51.
- While on night shift, you looked on the internet and read about heart-block. You are a bit worried that you may have damaged heart circuits, which may develop into 'heart-block'.

Your expectations:

- You expect to get an ECG, which you read about on the internet. You hope the GP can do it for you in surgery and hope you don't have to travel to the District Hospital, which is a nightmare to park at.
- If advised on lifestyle changes, ask specifically about "How much exercise?", or "What exactly is a healthy diet?" or "Is it OK to start exercising straight away?".

Medical history

You do not attend surgery very often. You do not have any allergies.

Social history

You are divorced. You met your current girlfriend through internet dating. You enjoy your social life and are proud of the recent lifestyle changes you made.

Information to reveal if examined

If the doctor asks to examine you:

- blood pressure: hand him/her a card saying "BP 136/84".
- pulse: regular 76bpm
- not anaemic
- normal heart sounds, no murmurs

SUGGESTED APPROACH TO THE CONSULTATION

Targeted history taking:

- What exactly does Neil mean by 'funny heartbeats'?

- For how long did the forceful and or irregular beats last? Elicit onset, intensity, duration, aggravating and relieving factors.

- Were there associated symptoms?

- Does he have risk factors for cardiac disease? Family history, smoking, high cholesterol, diabetes, or a sedentary lifestyle? Cause of anaemia? Thyroid symptoms? Exclude red flags, such as palpitations during exertion or palpitations with associated syncope or pre-syncope.

- What job does he do? What is his home life like?

- Is he going through a stressful time at the moment? Does he have a past history of anxiety?

- What does he think is the problem and its cause? Explore his family history.

- What are his expectations of this consultation: an examination, further investigation, a cardiology referral?

- What is his general health like – how much caffeine does he drink and how much exercise is he getting?

Targeted examination:

- A brief targeted CV examination is expected.

Clinical management:

- Reassure the patient that his symptoms (skipped beats, thumping beats, fluttering beats, slow pounding) usually point to benign palpitations. Palpitations associated with symptoms; palpitations associated with exercise; and palpitations associated with syncope/pre-syncope are more worrying.

- Discuss the natural history and aetiology of ectopics. The outlook is usually excellent and treatment is usually unnecessary.

- However, the patient's idea that his family history is significant is entirely valid. Even ventricular ectopics are sometimes a manifestation of sub-clinical heart disease and should therefore prompt general cardiac investigation (ECG, measurement of fasting glucose, cholesterol and/or TSH).

- Address the patient's concerns about having a significant arrhythmia such as heart block and perhaps provide more appropriate patient information, such as **Arrhythmia Alliance:** www.heartrhythmcharity.org.uk/

- Address the patient's expectations: arrange an ECG and blood tests.

- Provide brief lifestyle advice – stop smoking, more exercise and a healthier diet. Advise on reducing caffeine intake.
- Make follow-up arrangements.

Interpersonal skills:

This case tests the doctor's ability to explore what the patient means by 'funny heartbeats' and to gather sufficient data to decide on whether the patient requires GP investigation; routine (electrophysiology) OPD follow up; or urgent cardiology assessment. Data gathering needs to be systematic and the doctor needs to have sufficient knowledge to stratify the patient's risk to manage appropriately.

Good communication with the patient:

- elicits his concerns regarding an underlying cardiac problem.
- avoids lecturing the patient about his lifestyle.
- explores his expectations and negotiates appropriate investigation.
- provides an explanation about palpitations in a way which is understandable to him.
- gives targeted lifestyle advice and sets realistic goals in partnership with the patient.

Poor communication with the patient:

- does not elicit the reason for the patient's heightened anxiety, that is, his family history and his internet research.
- instructs the patient rather than mutually agrees goals.
- uses inappropriately technical language.
- is patronising or paternalistic in his reassurance.

BACKGROUND KNOWLEDGE REQUIRED FOR THIS CASE

Wolff, W and Cowan, C (2009) **10 steps before you refer for palpitations**.
Br. J. Cardiology, **16**: 182–6.

Palpitations could refer to heart racing but could mean a slow heart rate, an irregularity or an unusual pounding sensation; it is crucial to find out what patients actually mean.

Taking a family history:

- Are there any known cardiac conditions, such as heart muscle diseases, early onset atrial fibrillation and premature coronary disease, in close relatives?
- The use of an implantable cardioverter defibrillator (ICD) device in a young person might indicate an ion channel disease.

- Is there a family history of sudden cardiac death (SCD), especially deaths under the age of 40? It is advisable to ask a broad question: was there any unexplained sudden death in your family?
- As many as one in three patients with epilepsy are thought to be misdiagnosed. Many of those will suffer from reflex seizures instead, which can be caused by arrhythmic conditions. Therefore, a question on family history of epilepsy and sudden unexpected death in epilepsy (SUDEP) should be included.

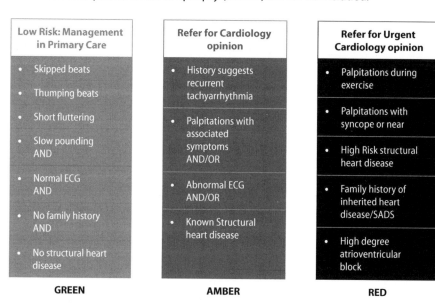

Low Risk: Management in Primary Care	Refer for Cardiology opinion	Refer for Urgent Cardiology opinion
• Skipped beats • Thumping beats • Short fluttering • Slow pounding AND • Normal ECG AND • No family history AND • No structural heart disease	• History suggests recurrent tachyarrhythmia • Palpitations with associated symptoms AND/OR • Abnormal ECG AND/OR • Known Structural heart disease	• Palpitations during exercise • Palpitations with syncope or near • High Risk structural heart disease • Family history of inherited heart disease/SADS • High degree atrioventricular block
GREEN	**AMBER**	**RED**

Risk stratification in arrhythmic illness using 'traffic light' system, proposed by Michael Cooklin. Available at: www.bradfordvts.co.uk/wp-content/onlineresources/1501cardiovascular/ palpitations%20in%20primary%20care.pdf

CASE 20 **Methotrexate**

INFORMATION FOR THE DOCTOR

This is a telephone consultation.

Name	George Thane
Age	41
Past medical history	• Psoriatic arthropathy 1 year ago • Psoriasis 3 years ago • Ganglion L wrist 10 years ago • Sciatica 11 years ago

The medical record of his **last consultation** 2 weeks ago, when he was seen by his usual GP, reads:

"Patient requests methotrexate repeat prescription – has been on 15mg once weekly (with folic acid 5mg once weekly) for seven months; no side-effects. Recent bloods (currently on monthly monitoring) show ALT is creeping up – now 70; rest fine. c/o sore throat so comes to have this examined.

O/E: throat normal. No cervical lymph nodes. T 36.1C HR 78 Oxygen sats 98%.

Plan – take meds as planned tonight but get repeat bloods in 2 weeks."

Current medication	• Methotrexate 2.5mg – 6 tablets once weekly • Folic acid 5mg once weekly • Betamethasone cream 0.1% apply twice daily • Calcipotriol cream apply once daily
Blood tests Hb Total WBC Platelets eGFR Creatinine Total bilirubin ALT* Alk Phos Alb CRP BMI Ex-smoker	*Blood tests done 2 days ago* 14.9g% (13–17) 6.91 (4–11) 301 (150–400) 90 82 (54–145) 11 (3–17) 136 (10–45) 131 (95–290) 46 (35–50) 0.7 (<11) 28

INFORMATION FOR THE PATIENT

You are George Thane, a 41-year-old heating engineer. You were diagnosed with psoriatic arthropathy seven months ago, after your GP referred you to Rheumatology with sore ankles and flitting pain in your left knee, right elbow, lower back and neck. You initially thought the pain was due to taking up running but when it failed to improve with rest, you Googled your symptoms and wondered if you had psoriatic arthropathy. You sometimes had swelling in your ankles and morning stiffness in the left ankle, which sometimes lasted as long as 30 minutes. The rheumatologist examined you, did blood tests and X-rays and diagnosed psoriatic arthropathy. They started you on methotrexate. You get the blood tests and repeat prescriptions from your GP under a shared care agreement. The blood monitoring has not picked up a problem before.

You have plaque psoriasis on your elbows and it is OK with the creams. Your nails have been pitted as well, which you understand is the psoriasis affecting the nails.

You are telephoning the GP today to discuss your blood results. You came two weeks ago because you were told if your throat was sore, you should have it examined. The doctor examined your throat and said you were OK to take the methotrexate but because your liver tests were not quite right, she wanted the blood tests repeated in two weeks' time, rather than in a month, which you think is a bit of an over-reaction. You telephone the surgery to discuss these results.

Your opening statement is *"I'm calling about my blood test, doctor. Is it OK to take my methotrexate tonight?"*.

Information to reveal if asked

General information about yourself:

- You are a self-employed heating engineer. You were scared when you started developing joint pain. You install and maintain boilers and need to be able to move equipment, sometimes into small spaces. Your GP and consultant told you that your joint problems were diagnosed quickly and that the methotrexate treatment would prevent the psoriasis from destroying the joint. Although you didn't like the sound of methotrexate (the patient leaflet lists many side-effects), you haven't had any problems and your joints seem a lot better. You are less worried about becoming riddled with painful arthritis and having to change jobs.

- Having never had a problem with methotrexate before, you don't think there's a big problem.

- You were told to lose weight, exercise more, and watch your alcohol intake. When first diagnosed, you restricted yourself to 2–4 pints of beer on weekends but recently you have been drinking a bit more.

- The psoriatic arthropathy diagnosis was a big shock. It scared you into thinking about your mortality. You have decided to work hard but also to enjoy life more. Hence you and your wife have planned a holiday to Kenya and Tanzania. Your wife is keen on doing a safari and watching the animal migration. You think the heat will help your joint ache and the sun will help your rash.

Further details about your condition:

- You now feel well, having completely recovered from your sore throat.
- You last saw the Rheumatologist 3 months ago and should see him again in 3 months' time.
- You have a book in which you wrote down your blood results, but the GPs and hospital doctors just checked results on the computer so you stopped using the book. You are not sure where this book is.

Your ideas:

- You think that the abnormal liver function tests a fortnight ago were a blip. You cut out alcohol completely before the repeat test 2 days ago.

Your concerns:

- You worry that if the liver tests come back as showing a problem, will you have to stop taking methotrexate? Could your arthritis get worse? Will you be put on other tablets? How will this affect your holiday, planned but not paid for, in 3 months' time?

Your expectations:

- You want to know what your blood tests showed.
- What do you do about methotrexate?
- When is the next blood test due?
- What should you tell your wife about Kenya?

Medical history

Since taking methotrexate, your skin psoriasis has cleared and you don't need to use the creams as often as you used to.

Social history

You are married. Your son is travelling on his gap year.

Information to reveal if examined

An examination is not needed.

SUGGESTED APPROACH TO THE CONSULTATION

Targeted history taking:

- What was the plan discussed at the last consultation? What medication is Mr Thane taking; at what dose; when was it last taken? Since the last dose, has he also taken any over-the-counter or complementary medication? Explore the alcohol history.

- Has methotrexate been effective and at what doses?

- When was the last review by the hospital and when is the next review due? Can he call a specialist nurse as part of his shared care? Does he have a written shared care agreement?

- Is he experiencing any other side-effects/any symptoms?

- Was he aware that methotrexate could have side-effects on the liver?

- What did he think about his recent results (especially the liver function) and ongoing use of medication?

- What information would he like from you today? If you are unable to give him the information now, what is the best way of contacting him later with this information?

Targeted examination:

- Not needed.

Clinical management:

- Discuss the latest blood results. ALT is above twice the upper level of normal. As neither you nor the patient have a copy of Shared Care Protocol to hand, either you or he need to call the Rheumatologist to decide on a management plan.

- Ask Mr Thane not to take any methotrexate until you obtain advice. You are likely to advise him to halve his dose of methotrexate and get a follow-up blood test in a week. He is likely to need regular blood tests (every 1–2 weeks) until his liver enzymes drop down to normal, after which the blood monitoring can go down to every two months. Hence over the next month, it may be better for him not to go on long overseas holidays.

- Mr Thane mentioned going to Kenya. Has he sought travel health advice (with the practice nurse/a travel health clinic) for the trip? Methotrexate is immunosuppressive and may therefore reduce immunological response to concurrent vaccination. Severe antigenic reactions may occur if a live vaccine is given concurrently. Mr Thane may want to check if vaccination is required for Kenya and Tanzania.

- Mr Thane mentioned how the diagnosis of psoriatic arthropathy was a life-changing event for him, leading to a shift in values. Discuss how he feels now.

Screen for depression and anxiety, assess quality of life, impact of symptoms on daily activities/work/relationships and family life.

- Manage the elevated liver enzymes and arrange appropriate follow-up, including screening for cardiovascular comorbidities if this has not previously been done.

Interpersonal skills:

Good communication with the patient:

- explores his current understanding and use of the prescribed medication.

- gives him time to comprehend the results and checks understanding.

- explores his health beliefs and treatment preferences in a sensitive and informed manner.

- negotiates and develops a shared plan with the patient; for example, about medication, CV screening and travel health advice.

BACKGROUND INFORMATION REQUIRED FOR THIS CASE

The British Society for Rheumatology (BSR) recommends precise monitoring to be carried out for methotrexate. The requirements are summarised as follows:

a. Pre-treatment assessment	FBC, U&E, LFTs, CXR
b. Ongoing monitoring	<ul><li>FBC fortnightly until 6 weeks after last dose increase</li><li>Provided it is stable, FBC monthly thereafter (may be reduced to every two months on advice from secondary care)</li><li>LFTs (incl. AST or ALT) with each blood test</li><li>U&Es 6–12 monthly (more frequently if there is any reason to suspect deteriorating renal function)</li></ul>
Additional monitoring not required but useful	ESR and/or CRP every three months

WBC <4 × 10⁹/L	Withhold until discussed with the specialist or his/her team
Neutrophils <2 × 10⁹/L	Withhold until discussed with the specialist or his/her team
Platelets <150 × 10⁹/L	Withhold until discussed with the specialist or his/her team
>2-fold rise in AST, ALT (from upper limit of reference range)	Withhold until discussed with the specialist or his/her team
Unexplained fall in albumin	Withhold until discussed with the specialist or his/her team
Rash or oral ulceration	Withhold until discussed with the specialist or his/her team
New or increasing dyspnoea or cough	Withhold until discussed with the specialist or his/her team
MCV >105fl	Investigate and if B12 or folate low, start appropriate supplementation
Significant deterioration in renal function	Reduce dose (discuss with the specialist or his/her team)
Abnormal bruising or sore throat	Withhold until FBC result available

Interactions:

- Do not prescribe co-trimoxazole (Septrin®) with methotrexate
- Other drugs which should be avoided include:
  - acitretin, chloramphenicol, sulphonamides, tetracyclines, thiazide diuretics, probenecid, sulfinpyrazone, oral hypoglycaemics, nitrous oxide and any drugs with suspected or confirmed hepatotoxic or nephrotoxic effects.
  - There are no contra-indications to using NSAIDs with doses of weekly methotrexate 25mg.

Weekly dosing of methotrexate is recommended. The entire dose can be administered at once. Methotrexate should never be given in daily doses. More frequent administration than weekly increases the risk of toxicity.

Most patients show a therapeutic response with weekly doses of oral or injection therapy between 7.5mg and 15.0mg, although some patients may need 20 or even 30mg, the maximum recommended dose.

Therapeutic response usually begins at 3 to 6 weeks, and the patient may continue to improve over a 12-week period.

For further information see:

www.aafp.org/afp/2000/1001/p1607.html

www.sign.ac.uk/pdf/sign121.pdf

CASE 21 **Postnatal/breast-feeding**

INFORMATION FOR THE DOCTOR

Name	Lauren Grey
Age	21
Past medical history	Tonsillectomy and adenoidectomy 7 years ago

The medical record of her **last consultation** 5 days ago (telephone call from duty doctor) reads:

"NVD 2 weeks ago. Tells me lost blood during delivery and was advised by midwife to get prescription for iron tablets. No problems with ferrous sulphate in past. Script issued. Advised to take tablets with orange juice. Advised on risk of constipation & diet. FBC booked."

Current medication	Ferrous sulphate 200mg, one tablet to be taken twice daily

INFORMATION FOR THE PATIENT

You are Lauren Grey, a 21-year-old single mum. You used to work as a nursery nurse but now intend to stay at home to look after your baby boy, Ethan. You have been breast-feeding exclusively (no bottles of formula milk or water) but Ethan is now feeding 'constantly'. His weight gain is slow, and Ethan has only just regained his birth weight. You are worried that your milk is not satisfying Ethan. He does not seem content or settled after feeds.

You are seeing the GP today because one of your friends told you there may be a tablet to help increase your milk production. Your mother advised you to give Ethan formula. If you switched to bottles, she said you'd sleep more and be less 'hormonal' during the day. You have been waking up at night to feed Ethan. He doesn't seem satisfied after feeding; he cries soon after feeding and wants to go back on the breast. You have been waking every two hours. You are tired. You have been getting upset over little things – you dropped a mug, it broke and you burst into tears. Your father commented on Ethan's clothes; you took this to be criticism and became "irrational". Your family think you have baby blues but you think you are tired.

Your opening statement is *"I don't want to, but I think I may have to put Ethan on formula milk. Is there an alternative, doctor?"*.

Information to reveal if asked

General information about yourself:

- Your relationship with Ethan's father did not work out and you do not intend to get back together with him. Ethan's dad texted to ask how you and Ethan were doing, but he had moved back to Scotland before Ethan's birth and has not seen Ethan. You do not expect him to keep in touch or make much effort to see Ethan. You have come to terms with this.

- Your mum and dad are supportive. Your mum works part-time and has provided practical and emotional support with Ethan.

- You love Ethan and you do not regret your decision to go ahead with the pregnancy despite pressure from Ethan's dad. You have bonded well with Ethan. You have found looking after him difficult. You worry about whether you are getting motherhood right.

Further details about your condition:

- You want to breast-feed. The midwife checked your feeding technique before you left hospital. Nobody has checked since. You think Ethan is latching on fine and while it 'yips' a little, the breast-feeding is pain free.

- If asked specifically, you describe how you breast-feed: Ethan is upright with his tummy to you; your breast is positioned to be opposite his nose; you move him to your breast and position him so you can see a bit of the areola above his top lip.

- You do not use a pacifier but if this crying persists, you intend to get one.
- If asked specifically, Ethan has 3–4 wet nappies per day and two stools per day. They are yellow, which you expected with breastfed babies.
- You are eating well and keeping healthy.

Your ideas:

- You think you need a tablet to help you to make more breast milk.
- You think that your mood swings and irritability are due to your hormones and tiredness. You have feelings of despondency and anxiety but you do enjoy things, you have an appetite and if given the chance, you sleep well and feel refreshed.

Your concerns:

- You do not want to 'fail at breast-feeding' and it would feel like failing to switch to bottles. You think that breast-feeding is helping Ethan's immunity and giving him a good start in life. You are concerned that the doctor will advise you to give Ethan formula, 'for his own good' or 'fob you off' to the Health Visitor who cannot prescribe tablets.

Your expectations:

- You want a prescription for tablets to help with breast milk production.

Medical history

You are healthy. You have an allergy to shellfish.

Social history

You are not currently in a relationship. Your relationship with Ethan's dad is over but you are disappointed that he has not made an effort to see his son.

You do not smoke. You have the occasional glass of alcohol; not much now because of the pregnancy and breast-feeding.

Information to reveal if examined

You are not depressed or anxious.

SUGGESTED APPROACH TO THE CONSULTATION

Targeted history taking:

- Why does Lauren think that her milk is not satisfying Ethan? Could Ethan have problems attaching or feeding, such as tongue tie?

- How often is she feeding, is she offering supplementary feeds, what is her feeding technique, does she experience any symptoms while feeding?

- Is she taking on board adequate food and water?

- Is she using medication such as combined hormonal contraception that could be reducing her milk supply?

- Is there evidence of insufficient milk intake in Ethan: fewer than 6 wet nappies per 24 hours; fewer than 3 stools per day; persistent jaundice; slow or no weight gain?

- Explore whether Lauren is tired or depressed. What support does she have?

- What does Lauren think is contributing to her reduced milk production and what does she think would be a good solution?

- Is there anything in particular that is worrying Lauren, such as Ethan being unwell, or whether she is doing 'something wrong'?

- What would Lauren like you to do for her?

Targeted examination:

- Briefly assess her mood.

Clinical management:

- Lauren is understandably concerned: Ethan is having <6 wet nappies per day, producing less than 3 stools per day, and is not settled or contented after feeds, which are signs of insufficient milk intake.

- Having explored that Lauren's breast-feeding technique is good, encourage more frequent skin-to-skin contact, breast massage and nipple stimulation to stimulate more milk production.

- Consider whether expressed milk could be given between feeds.

- Discuss medication such as domperidone, which is used 'off-label'.

- If prescribing domperidone, use 10–20mg TDS or QDS. Advise that an increase in milk production is seen in 3–4 days. However, it may take 2–3 weeks to see the full effect. Domperidone use can be discontinued once milk production is optimised, usually within 3–8 weeks.

- Arrange follow-up to check for problems with medication and to review mood, to check if better sleep improves tiredness, mood swings and irritability.

Interpersonal skills:

This case tests the doctor's ability to assess two intertwined issues: reduced breast milk production and post-natal mood issues. By taking a good and systematic history of the baby's symptoms (number of wet and soiled nappies, etc.), the doctor is able to diagnose a serious feeding problem. The danger here is to be diverted by the mood symptoms before carefully assessing the feeding. If the feeding is not recognised and managed, mum could resort to formula in desperation. By considering domperidone, the doctor considers the pros and cons of (1) off-label prescribing with (2) switching to formula milk. The doctor and patient then develop a shared management plan.

Good communication with the patient:

- uses specific closed questions after the open exploratory questions to assess the severity of the feeding problem.
- assesses mood, sleep, bonding and ability to control behaviour despite swings in mood and feelings.
- summarises the problem and diagnosis.
- offers treatment options, and is able to explain off-label prescribing.
- is supportive to a struggling and tired young mum.

Poor communication with the patient:

- is haphazard and unsystematic in data gathering, or makes assumptions without clarifying details.
- deviates, with little justification, from the patient's agenda.
- fails to offer treatment options, or explain off-label prescribing or facilitate patient choice.

BACKGROUND KNOWLEDGE REQUIRED FOR THIS CASE

NHMRC, Australia (2012) **Infant feeding guidelines**.

Mothers can be reassured regarding the adequacy of their milk volume and quality if the infant:

- is fully breastfed – that is, receiving no other fluids or solids – and producing **six to eight very wet nappies** of pale, inoffensive-smelling urine in a 24-hour period.
- has **appropriate weight gain** when averaged out over a 4-week period, remembering that infants often lose 5–10% of their birth weight during the first week. Weight gain in the 1st three months is expected at 150–200g per week.
- produces stool, which can be loose/runny and mustard-coloured, with a few days between stools. Dry hard stool that is painful to pass is of concern.

- is **alert**, with bright eyes, moist lips and good skin tone and
- is reasonably **content** for some time between some feeds.

Physiological jaundice develops on day 2–4 and clears by the second week. Persistent or deep jaundice is of concern.

Strategies to ensure adequate milk supply

- Check positioning and attachment
- Feed more frequently – offer the breast between the usual feeds; offer the breast as a comforter instead of a pacifier
- Wake the infant and offer an extra feed before going to bed
- Allow the infant to finish the first breast before offering the second breast
- Always feed from each breast more than once each feed
- Express milk between feeds.

Management:

- Recommend a healthy, well-balanced diet
- Discourage excessive exercise and weight-loss diets
- Ensure adequate fluid intake by encouraging the mother to drink a glass of water every time she breast-feeds and when thirsty
- Encourage rest and relaxation
- Suggest frequent skin-to-skin contact, breast massage and nipple stimulation.

Galactogogues (substances that promote breast milk supply) include metoclopramide, domperidone and recombinant human prolactin. These drugs have not been approved for use as galactogogues and use would be 'off-label'.

Relevant literature

www.breastfeedingnetwork.org.uk/wp-content/dibm/BfN%20statement%20on%20domperidone%20as%20a%20galactogogue.pdf

CASE 22 Recurrent nipple pain

INFORMATION FOR THE DOCTOR

Name	Harriet Grant
Age	35
Past medical history	• Mastitis 3 months ago • Normal vaginal delivery 8 months ago • Anaemia during pregnancy 10 months ago • Hyperemesis 15 months ago • Normal vaginal delivery 3 years ago • Sprained ankle 11 years ago

The medical record of her **last consultation** in surgery 3 months ago (when she was seen by usual GP) reads:

"3 weeks ago had thrush on nipples and son had oral thrush. Settled with topical anti-fungal. Few days ago c/o redness and soreness R breast outer lower quadrant. Patient says she had thrush in milk ducts with last baby and it needed oral anti-fungals.
O/E: R breast outer lower quadrant – red, hot, lumpy with disproportionate tenderness. L breast NAD.
Plan – looks more like mastitis. Pros and cons of antibiotics versus anti-fungals discussed. Opts for antibiotics. Offered to review next week, sooner if problems."

Current medication	• Flucloxacillin 500mg QDS for 7 days • Canesten HC cream 1% apply twice daily
Blood tests Hb Total WBC MCV MCH	*Blood tests done 10 months ago* 11.5g% (13–17) 8.33 (4–11) 90 (85–105) 30.3 (27–32)
BMI Non-smoker Not in date with smear	25

INFORMATION FOR THE PATIENT

You are Harriet Grant, a 35-year-old stay at home mother of two. You were diagnosed with mastitis of the right breast 3 months ago, took a week of antibiotic tablets which helped for a while and then symptoms recurred. You were concerned when you saw the GP 3 months ago about having intra-ductal fungal infection and you were surprised to be told you had mastitis.

The GP asked you to see the Health Visitor (HV) to check your breastfeeding technique. The HV, having observed you, felt your breastfeeding technique was good. Despite the antibiotics, good breastfeeding technique, OTC anti-fungal cream, lanolin and E45 you have a recurrence of nipple symptoms.

Both nipples are affected. The nipples over a period of 2–4 days have become sore, red, and cracked. The discomfort becomes quite painful (5/10) with breastfeeding. The pain intensifies with latching on and remains constant throughout the feed. Between feeds, it is uncomfortable (not painful), and sometimes itchy.

You are seeing the GP today to get treatment for recurrent thrush. When you treat the 'nipple thrush', it goes away, but when you stop treatment, it comes back. Your little boy has some white patches on the left inner cheek which you think is oral thrush. He was treated with nystatin in the past. His feeding has never been affected; he feeds well.

Your opening statement is *"I think I have nipple thrush again, doctor. I'm a bit run down"*.

Information to reveal if asked

General information about yourself:

- You are a 35-year-old full-time mum. You are very busy with two boys, playgroups, swimming and church activities.
- You have had about 6 episodes of nipple pain with this baby, but only came to the GP on two occasions; one diagnosed as thrush and the other as mastitis.
- You had eczema affecting your elbows and knees as a child.
- You do not have a family history of psoriasis, skin cancer or breast cancer.

Further details about your condition:

- You feel well, not flu-like and do not have temperature symptoms.
- Sometimes there is a white fluid substance between the nipple folds, like a discharge, but no pus and no yellow crusting. Sometimes there are flaky white scales. Sometimes the nipples crack. It has not bled. It can be itchy.

- The symptoms today are confined to your nipples. They usually are. The breast was affected on the last occasion when mastitis was diagnosed.
- Your son is eating baby food and only has 3 or 4 small feeds (3 ounces you think) per feed. You want to breastfeed until he is one year old. You do not want to express milk or use a bottle.
- Your son is biting hard substances and drooling but he does not have any baby teeth.

Your ideas:

- You think this is thrush because you had something similar in your last pregnancy which disappeared with anti-fungal tablets. OTC Canesten HC helped but did not prevent recurrence.
- Your symptoms get worse after antibiotics or when you are run down. This bout came on after a recent severe cold.

Your concerns:

- You worry about recurrent thrush. With two young boys at playgroups and nursery, you are forever getting colds and coughs. When you are run down, your symptoms flare. You are concerned about getting recurrent minor illnesses that your boys will bring home from playgroups and school.

Your expectations:

- You want a prescription.
- You want some advice on how to reduce the recurrence. Should you be taking something to boost your immunity?

Medical history

The doctor gave you iron tablets in your pregnancy but your midwife thought that was unnecessary. You did not lose a large amount of blood with your deliveries.

Social history

You are happily married.

Information to reveal if examined

Decline a chaperone.

Hand the doctor a picture of your nipples (to show them the picture on your phone, go to www.dermnetnz.org/site-age-specific/lactation.html and see image 2).

SUGGESTED APPROACH TO THE CONSULTATION

Targeted history taking:

- What are Mrs Grant's symptoms? Clarify if she has nipple or breast pain; nipple or breast skin changes; discharge; and/or systemic symptoms.

- Take a history of the pain: nature; duration; periodicity, associated symptoms. Does the pain change as she breastfeeds? What makes the pain worse and what helps improve the pain?

- Take a history of the discharge: duration, frequency, volume and colour of nipple discharge and whether it occurs spontaneously or only on feeding; whether bilateral. Has she ever felt a lump?

- Does Mrs Grant have a history of breast or skin problems? How is today's presentation different to previous presentations? What has helped and not helped in the past?

- What does she think is causing the pain? What are her reasons for thinking this?

- What is she worried about? Is she concerned about infection, or cancer or 'being run down'? What are the possible causes for her being 'run down' and could she be anaemic?

- What does Mrs Grant want from this consultation: a prescription, advice, a check of her breastfeeding technique, advice on the 'white spots' in her little boy's mouth?

- Does Mrs Grant have any allergies; is her skin easily irritated by anything?

Targeted examination:

- Ask to examine her breasts and whether she wants a chaperone present.

- Mrs Grant hands you a picture: see *Background medical knowledge required for this case*.

Clinical management:

- Summarise the main findings from history and examination.

- Discuss the findings – red, scaling, cracked, painful nipples (and areolar skin) in a patient with a history of atopic eczema may be nipple eczema. The skin may be irritated by the trauma of breastfeeding, or food particles from the infant's mouth, or bacteria entering the milk ducts. This could be an 'eczema flare'. Fungal infection is often over-diagnosed, but is possible particularly if the baby has oral thrush, but could the baby's symptoms be attributed to teething and trauma to the inner cheek?

- Discuss treatment of an eczema flare: antibiotic creams, steroid ointments, emollients.

- Explore the reasons for feeling 'run down' and assess whether a FBC and/or ferritin level is needed.

- Mrs Grant mentioned the Health Visitor had checked her feeding technique. If the skin is being irritated by food particles or just the trauma of normal latching on, how does Mrs Grant wish to deal with it?

- Arrange appropriate follow-up. There should be a response to steroid ointment if the diagnosis was correct.

Interpersonal skills:

This case tests the doctor's ability to systematically explore a presenting complaint and reach his or her own differential diagnosis. The doctor should be able to consider the reasons for and against various differentials: eczema, psoriasis, nipple hypersensitivity, bacterial or fungal infection, nipple vasospasm, mastitis or Paget's disease of the nipple. The patient offers up a diagnosis, namely fungal infection. However, the doctor needs to explore the symptoms that have led the patient to believe she may have a fungal infection and consider if there are alternative explanations for these symptoms. The doctor with good interpersonal skills is able to negotiate the agenda without seeming patronising. For example, in response to Mrs Grant's opening statement that she has nipple thrush again, the doctor could say "You know Mrs Grant, when someone says they have something 'again', a small alarm bell goes off in my head. Either I have to discover why they are getting it again, or I have to see if we got the diagnosis right. So tell me more about your symptoms."

Good communication with the patient:

- explores her symptoms – are these the symptoms and signs of a nipple fungal infection or eczema flare?

- explores her health beliefs and explores why she may be 'run down'.

- establishes her preferences for treatment – negotiates medication and discusses what she would like to do about breastfeeding.

- explores her understanding of the diagnosis and treatment plan offered – a good 'handover' occurs

- negotiates follow-up – 'safety-nets'.

Therefore, once the patient's ideas, concerns and expectations have been elicited, and the clinical priorities negotiated, the management plan is developed in true partnership with the patient.

BACKGROUND KNOWLEDGE REQUIRED FOR THIS CASE

- Some common skin problems, particularly of the nipple, areola and breast, may appear during breastfeeding.

- An underlying skin condition, such as atopic eczema or psoriasis, may contribute to this.

- Poor breastfeeding techniques may also precipitate or aggravate skin problems.

- In addition to treating the skin complaint, women are also likely to need support and advice with regard to breastfeeding.

- Nipple hypersensitivity is common during the first postpartum week. Usually this peaks at day 3–6 and then subsides.

- Pain in the first two weeks postpartum is most commonly due to trauma to the nipple secondary to poor breastfeeding technique.

- A nipple suction injury that does not heal with a change in breastfeeding technique may be a sign of infection, usually with *Staphylococcus aureus*.

- Postpartum women can have increased skin sensitivity to environmental irritants and those with an atopic history can present with an eczema flare. Topical corticosteroids are the main treatment. They should be applied sparingly after a breastfeed. Ointments are preferred to creams.

- Vasospasm in the vessels of the nipple results in colour change in the nipple and stabbing shooting pain. Vasospasm is often triggered by an initial injury to the nipple but may also be a response to cold or a manifestation of Raynaud phenomenon.

Relevant literature

Neighbour, R. (2004) *The Inner Consultation*, 2nd edition. Radcliffe Medical Press.

For further information see:

www.dermnetnz.org/site-age-specific/lactation.html (nipple eczema – image 2)

www.pcds.org.uk/clinical-guidance/atopic-eczema

CASE 23 UTI

INFORMATION FOR THE DOCTOR

Name	Chioma Uwak
Age	27
Social and family history	• Divorced, no children • Cigarette smoker (15 cig/day) • Alcohol 10 units/week
Past medical history	• Suspected UTI – nitrofurantoin prescribed 2 months ago • Cystitis – trimethoprim prescribed 3 months ago • Breakthrough bleeding on POP 2 years ago Negative for chlamydia • Focal migraines on combined pills 12 years ago
Current medication	• Cerazette 1 tablet daily × 168T • Mefenamic acid 500mg twice daily PRN, for breakthrough bleeding
Clinical values BMI BP Smear	*Tests done 2 years ago* 21 114/64 Normal

INFORMATION FOR THE PATIENT

You are Chioma Uwak, a 27-year-old catering assistant, who has come to discuss your urinary symptoms. Over the last 24 hours, you have been passing small amounts of urine, every 2–3 hours and it really hurts to urinate. You think you passed blood last night, but this could have been breakthrough bleeding from your mini-Pill.

You present to the doctor expecting to get antibiotics for your cystitis. Your opening statement is *"I think I've got another urine infection"*.

Information to reveal if asked

General information about yourself:

- You work for a catering firm. You help with some food preparation, but mainly you set up the dining area and serve the food at events.

- You started a new sexually active relationship 3 months ago. You stopped using condoms 2 months ago. You thought the latex may be predisposing you to developing urine infections. You were OK for 2 months but then you developed symptoms again yesterday.

- You work with your partner. He is a chef. He broke up with his girlfriend 4 months ago because she was unfaithful. He told you he had STI tests at the clinic and was 'clear'. You are asymptomatic and have not had any STI tests since the doctor checked for chlamydia when you had some spotting on the mini-Pill a couple of years ago.

- You smoke 10 cigarettes per day. You are thinking of trying electronic cigarettes but you enjoy smoking. Your new partner smokes.

- You enjoy a beer or 1–2 glasses of wine 3–4 times per week.

- You used to get migraines when you had periods but you tend not to get periods on your mini-Pill and haven't had a migraine for a few years.

Further details about your condition:

- You have lower abdominal discomfort.

- You do not have temperature symptoms. You do not have nausea or vomiting.

- You have leaked small amounts of urine by not getting to the toilet on time.

- You get urine symptoms when sexually active. Usually drinking cranberry juice or drinking lots of water gets rid of the symptoms so you don't see a doctor for antibiotics.

Your ideas:

- You think that you have honeymoon cystitis but you have been scared by the blood, which you are not sure is from the urine or from the breakthrough bleeding on the mini-Pill.

- In the past, you were treated with antibiotics which helped. You did not have side-effects.

- One doctor asked for a urine sample and did a test in surgery. You don't think the urine was ever sent to the hospital for testing.

- You don't think you have a sexually transmitted disease and you don't want to be tested.

- If the doctor offers to do a urine test, you say you have just been to the bathroom and can't pass any urine just now. You can drop a sample off later, on your way to work.

Your concerns:

- You are worried about not being given antibiotics. You need to work over the next few nights and tips tend to be generous at this venue.

- You have had a few infections and are wondering why you seem to get urine infections after sex so often.

Your expectations:

- You expect to get some antibiotics. You didn't have a problem with the antibiotics previously prescribed and don't have a preference for a particular antibiotic.

Medical history

You are happy on the mini-Pill and do not wish to change contraception. You do not want to see a smoking cessation nurse at present.

Social history

You are enjoying your current relationship.

Information to reveal if examined

If the doctor asks to examine your abdomen, give him/her a card saying "supra-pubic discomfort only".

SUGGESTED APPROACH TO THE CONSULTATION

Targeted history taking:

- What are Chioma's symptoms now? How did the symptoms start? Any precipitating events? How did the symptoms evolve? Did she try anything (such as cranberry) to ease the symptoms? What was the effect?

- Has she had nausea, vomiting, fevers, back pain or vaginal discharge in addition to haematuria or PV bleeding? Has she been able to keep her contraceptive tablet down? Could she be pregnant?

- Has she had urine infections in the past? Has she had urine tests or any scans done?

- Why does she think she is getting so many urine infections in such a short period of time?

- What are her concerns? Is she worried that an underlying medical issue (which predisposes her to UTIs) is being overlooked?

- What are her expectations: does she expect medication and specific advice to reduce recurrence?

- How does she feel about 'stand-by' antibiotics or cranberry prophylaxis?

Targeted examination:

- This case does not require the candidate to perform a targeted physical examination.

Clinical management:

- Chioma is a non-pregnant young woman with frequency and dysuria. She does not have vaginal discharge, low back pain or temperature symptoms. You can make a diagnosis of bacterial UTI.

- Discuss the management of bacterial UTI.

- Discuss what Chioma should do if symptoms do not resolve after 3 days – bring an MSU to send for MC&S to guide further antibiotic prescribing, based on resistance patterns.

- Address the patient's ideas: that she has honeymoon cystitis – 2 or more UTIs in 6 months, or 3 or more UTIs in 12 months provoked by sex. Discuss how this may be treated either with self-initiated antibiotics (3 days trimethoprim or nitrofurantoin) or post-coital antibiotics 100mg trimethoprim or 100mg nitrofurantoin post-coitally. Alternatively, prophylactic OTC cranberry products, such as capsules or juice, could be used.

- Address the patient's concerns about this infection not being treated promptly with antibiotics. You do not have to send a sample of urine off for lab testing.

Based on her symptoms, you may prescribe empirically. She is worried about recurrent UTIs provoked by sex. Unfortunately this is not an uncommon occurrence, hence the advice about post-coital antibiotics or keeping a course of antibiotics at home to start as soon as symptoms of frequency and dysuria occur.

- Address the patient's expectations for antibiotics – prescribe a 3-day course of trimethoprim or nitrofurantoin. Take steps to promote concordance.

- Confirm her understanding of bacterial UTIs, honeymoon cystitis and the treatment options for this. Discuss how patients could tell the difference between UTI, pyelonephritis and STIs.

- Safety-net – discuss when and why she should consult again.

Interpersonal skills:

This case tests the doctor's ability to take a straightforward history and manage a simple case. Most candidates are thrown by a simple case, expecting there to be a hidden agenda. If you have established rapport with the patient and created a space in which the patient feels comfortable to reveal information, and if the patient answers no to your question *'is there anything else I can help you with?'* then trust the data-gathering and move on. Constantly fishing for a hidden agenda is likely to annoy the patient and waste time.

Good communication with the patient:

- addresses the patient's agenda regarding honeymoon cystitis.

- empathises with her problem and discusses without embarrassment bacterial UTIs provoked by sex.

- is respectful and non-judgemental – offers but does not insist on STI testing or smoking cessation advice.

- explains the immediate and long-term treatment options clearly and answers any questions the patient has.

- respects her treatment preferences.

- safety-nets appropriately.

BACKGROUND KNOWLEDGE REQUIRED FOR THIS CASE

SIGN (2012) **Management of suspected UTIs in adults**. http://www.sign.ac.uk/pdf/sign88.pdf

Women with symptomatic LUTI should receive empirical antibiotic treatment.

Use dipstick tests to guide treatment decisions in otherwise healthy women under 65 years of age presenting with mild or ≤2 symptoms of UTI.

Consider empirical treatment with an antibiotic for otherwise healthy women aged less than 65 years of age presenting with severe or ≥3 symptoms of UTI. If dysuria and frequency are both present, then the probability of UTI is increased to >90% and empirical treatment with antibiotic is indicated.

If vaginal discharge is present, the probability of bacteriuria falls. Alternative diagnoses such as sexually transmitted diseases (STDs) and vulvovaginitis, usually due to candida, are likely and pelvic examination is indicated.

Treat non-pregnant women of any age with symptoms or signs of acute LUTI with a three-day course of trimethoprim or nitrofurantoin. Take urine for culture to guide change of antibiotic for patients who do not respond to trimethoprim or nitrofurantoin.

Evidence from a controlled before and after study (CBA) and an RCT showed that telephone consultation by nurse practitioners is as effective and safe as standard consultation in a medical practitioner's office, is preferred by a majority of women and is likely to be cost saving.

There is good evidence to support prevention of recurrent bacterial UTI in women with antibiotics and cranberry products. These strategies should be explored before referral for specialist investigation.

CASE 24 Heel pain

INFORMATION FOR THE DOCTOR

Name	Miles Beckett
Age	28
Social and family history	Married, one child age 8 weeks
Past medical history	Insurance medical for mortgage 2 years ago – nil of note
Acute medication	Ibuprofen 400mg thrice daily × 84 tablets

The medical record of his **last consultation** by Dr Brown (three weeks ago) reads:

"Actuary with gradual onset (4 weeks) L heel pain, worse medially. Started with morning pain and worse after activity. Now unable to finish rugby game over weekend because of 8/10 pain – walked off field. O/E: tender anterior to heel. Impression: typical plantar fasciitis. Plan: ibuprofen × 84T and refer to physiotherapy." (However, there is no referral letter attached to the consultation).

INFORMATION FOR THE PATIENT

You are Miles Beckett, a 28-year-old actuary, who has come to the doctor to find out what happened to your physiotherapy appointment. When you called the physiotherapy unit to initiate an appointment, they informed you that they hadn't received a GP referral letter. You want to know what happened.

You have also come for advice. Your foot still hurts despite rest, ice and ibuprofen for three weeks and you want alternative medication or 'something different'. You were informed by one of your rugby colleagues that an X-ray may be needed to see if you have a heel spur. Should you have an X-ray?

If the doctor does not offer you a suitable explanation or apology for what happened to your referral, you become increasingly distrustful, irritated and overtly dissatisfied by what you perceive to be a 'shoddy' service. If the doctor offers you a private referral to reduce waiting times, you inform the doctor that you do not have private insurance but will be happy to take up the offer if the practice will pay for it as they inadvertently delayed your treatment. If the doctor offers you a follow-up appointment in the surgery for a steroid injection, you ask about risks and benefits and choose not to have this done without trying non-invasive treatments first. If the doctor gives you advice that will help you while you wait for your NHS physiotherapy appointment, you leave feeling 'something has been done to move things in the right direction' and appear slightly appeased.

You present to the doctor expecting to discuss what happened to your physiotherapy appointment and for alternative treatment as rest and ibuprofen did not work. Your opening statement is *"The physio chaps say they didn't get a referral and my heel pain is still pretty bad"*.

Information to reveal if asked
General information about yourself:

- You work in the city centre, commuting in to work by train. This is a busy service and usually you have to stand for 20 minutes before you can get a seat. The heel starts to ache after standing on it for too long.

- You are married with 1 child, aged 8 weeks. Baby Poppy wakes at night and you help to bottle-feed. You find the night walking, with baby in arms, painful.

- You have never been ill before and are worried about your foot. You assumed you would make a quick recovery once you rested the foot for a couple of weeks and completed a course of ibuprofen.

Further details about your condition:

- The left heel pain started about two months ago and Dr Brown thought it was plantar fasciitis which you understand to be inflammation where a thick bit of tissue in your foot attaches to the heel.

- The pain is worse when you first stand, or walk, or run, and then seems to improve as the foot warms and loosens up. It is worse if you walk in slippers or flip-flops, which you use when you walk Poppy at night. Running shoes are the most comfortable footwear.

- Some of your friends at the rugby club are considering a running challenge in the New Year, to run as many miles as there are in the year, so a total of 2017 miles run over the course of 2017. You, as a rugby winger, would like to do something like this before you are thirty and don't want to pull out as an 'old crock'.

Your ideas:

- You think that your foot pain is plantar fasciitis, but you are disappointed that rest, icing with frozen peas and regular ibuprofen made no difference at all. If asked specifically, the intensity of the pain when you first put weight on the foot has reduced. If you walk in running shoes rather than slippers, the pain is less. However, you cannot walk fast or run and you still get heel pain if you stand for too long on the train.

- You think physiotherapy will help. You spoke to a club physiotherapist who was providing medical cover at a game and she said you'll need to be assessed before the right exercises can be prescribed. However, she only provides emergency not routine treatment at the club so she can't treat you.

- You feel that your tax and National Insurance contributions help fund the health service. You feel that you don't have to pay more for private healthcare.

- You would like to use the NHS. You feel the NHS is a good thing but you don't like inefficiency and poor service. However, you understand that mistakes can be made and if the doctor admits that a mistake has been made and apologises for the delay in your care, then you are prepared to accept the apology.

Your concerns:

- You are worried about the length of time it is taking for the problem to heal and whether 'stronger' tablets should be given or something different should be tried.

- You are also worried about whether the diagnosis is correct – should you have an X-ray to rule out a foot fracture (you have heard about stress fractures in athletes) or a heel spur (which your rugby mate has mentioned to you)?

- You suspect that you may not be up for the long distance running challenge, which is annoying.

Your expectations:

- You expect to get information about the missing physiotherapy referral and have a discussion about X-ray investigation and treatment of heel pain.

Medical history

You consider yourself to be fit. You occasionally binge drink on weekends, but overall lead a much healthier life now. You do not currently have any side effects from the ibuprofen.

Social history

You are happily married and Poppy is a delightful baby, but it does take some walking and back rubbing after a feed to settle her back to sleep.

Information to reveal if examined

If the doctor asks to examine your feet, you are tender in front of the left heel. When walking, the medial arch (observed from behind), drops creating a flat foot that rolls in.

You are not overweight.

See www.sportsinjuryclinic.net/sport-injuries/foot-heel-pain/plantar-fasciitis/plantar-fasciitis-diagnosis

SUGGESTED APPROACH TO THE CONSULTATION

Targeted history taking:

- When was the referral supposed to have been done and is there any evidence that the referral left the practice?

- What are Miles's symptoms now? What was his response to the rest and anti-inflammatories? Did he experience any side-effects from the anti-inflammatories?

- What does he suspect is causing his left heel pain? What's leading him to these conclusions? What does he understand about the natural history and treatment of plantar fasciitis?

- What are his concerns? Is he worried that the diagnosis is correct and whether X-ray will help to make the diagnosis? Is he worried about ongoing treatment and how helpful that may be in 'curing' the problem?

- What would he like you to do – investigate the missing physiotherapy referral, apologise, discuss alternative treatments, re-refer?

- Is he prepared to consider analgesia, relative rest, steroid injections, frictional massage or a self-help leaflet on stretching and strengthening exercises?

Targeted examination:

- This case does not require the candidate to perform a targeted physical examination because the history and examination findings of the previous consultation are so typical of plantar fasciitis. No new information is revealed in today's discussion that prompts the doctor to examine the foot again.

Clinical management:

- Having read the patient information provided prior to the consultation, be alerted by the absence of a referral letter.

- Summarise back to the patient the pertinent issues (missing physiotherapy referral, concern over correct diagnosis and ongoing left heel pain) and empathise with Mr Beckett's feelings of anxiety and frustration. For example, the doctor could say *"The absence of a referral letter both at the physiotherapy department and here in your notes does not look too promising, does it? I can see how you could be feeling worried about being let down. I don't know what has happened, but I promise you I will look into it and try to resolve this as best I can. Either way, your treatment has been delayed and for that, I apologise. Now, I haven't seen you before so I need to ask you some questions so that I can help you"*.

- Address the patient's expectation regarding whether the diagnosis of plantar fasciitis is correct by clarifying details about current symptoms and response to rest and NSAIDs. Explore red flags by asking about morning stiffness, back and buttock pain, and tenderness in ligament insertions in the extremities (symptoms of Reiter's disease or ankylosing spondylitis because a small minority of these patients present with plantar fasciitis). This set of questions could be signposted by saying, *"To rule out serious illness I need to ask you a few quick questions. Are your joints stiff in the morning?; do you have pain in the…?"*.

- Confirm a working diagnosis of plantar fasciitis based on the typical history.

- Mr Beckett's idea that PF resolves quickly may be optimistic. Studies show that most cases resolve by 6 to 12 months. 5% of patients end up undergoing surgery for plantar fascia release when conservative measures fail (see http://emedicine.medscape.com/article/86143-treatment).

- Negotiate physiotherapy referral. You could offer to add in a paragraph explaining that the patient had consulted 3 weeks ago and the original referral is missing. You could ask Mr Beckett if he could be available for short notice appointments if other patients cancel and indicate his availability and/or flexibility on the referral document.

- Address his expectations for practical advice: discuss footwear, orthotics, silicone heel pads, steroid injections, self-massage by rolling the foot on a golf ball, stretching and strengthening exercises (see http://www.aafp.org/afp/20010201/467.html). Advise discontinuation of NSAIDs beyond 10 days and consider alternative analgesia. As Mr Beckett has a good basic understanding of PF, build on this knowledge by discussing exercises (foot biomechanics) and self-help treatments.

- Provide some information on the pros and cons of steroid injection, but discuss the potential risks of rupture of the plantar fascia and fat pad atrophy.

- Provide information on X-rays: PF produces heel spurs; heel spurs do not produce PF. Hence, the spur, if present, should not be surgically removed. An X-ray may not add to the management. The history is not really suggestive of a stress fracture.

Interpersonal skills:

This case tests the doctor's ability to deal with a verbal complaint and consult with an (understandably) aggrieved patient. The good candidate is able to acknowledge and empathise with the patient's feeling *before* moving on to the business end of the consultation.

Good communication involves:

- establishing rapport by listening attentively to Mr Beckett's opening statements and acknowledging his feelings of fear, anxiety and frustration.

- dealing with his anger at the 'lost' referral without placing undue blame on other members of staff.

- displaying empathy to the duration of illness and its adverse consequences.

- addressing the patient's specific concerns and expectations and encouraging self-help.

- encouraging autonomy and opinions – providing him with treatment options, discussing their risks and benefits and facilitating the patient's choice.

- Good prescribing behaviour involves discussing how NSAIDs should be used in a chronic condition such as PF and discussing alternative analgesia.

BACKGROUND KNOWLEDGE REQUIRED FOR THIS CASE

Young, CC *et al.* (2001) **Treatment of plantar fasciitis.** *American Family Physician,* **63(3)**: 467–475.
http://www.aafp.org/afp/20010201/467.html

The classic sign of plantar fasciitis is that the worst pain occurs with the first few steps in the morning, but not every patient will have this symptom. Patients often notice pain at the beginning of activity that lessens or resolves as they warm up.

A history of an increase in weight-bearing activities is common, especially those involving running, which causes microtrauma to the plantar fascia.

Plantar fasciitis is a self-limiting condition, often taking 6 to 18 months, which can lead to frustration for patients and physicians. Rest is often the treatment that works best, or "relative rest" in athletic patients who substitute alternative forms of activity (cross-training or cycling) for activities (hard walking or running) that aggravate the symptoms.

Stretching and strengthening programmes are important to correct functional risk factors such as tightness of the gastrocsoleus complex and weakness of the intrinsic foot muscles. Increasing flexibility of the calf muscles is particularly important.

One RCT found arch taping and orthotics were significantly better than use of NSAIDs, cortisone injection or heel cups.

CASE 25 Grief

INFORMATION FOR THE DOCTOR

Name	Aisha Chetty
Age	54
Social and family history	Married, three adult children
Past medical history	Hypercholesterolaemia for 3 years
Current medication	Atorvastatin 10mg daily (on last issue of repeat prescription)
Blood tests Plasma fasting glucose Fasting cholesterol Fasting HDL cholesterol Total cholesterol:HDL Alkaline phosphatase Total bilirubin Albumin Creatinine level	*Blood tests done 13 months ago* 5.4mmol/L (3.65–5.5) 5.1mmol/L 1.4mmol/L (0.8–1.8) 3.6 164IU/L (95–280) 17µmol/L (3–17) 39g/L (35–50) 102µmol/L (70–150)
BMI BP	26 138/82

INFORMATION FOR THE PATIENT

You are Aisha Chetty, a 54-year-old post office worker, who has come to discuss your current emotional distress. You want 'something to help' with your grief. You are weepy and 'shocked'.

Your sister-in-law had a fatal MI in India three weeks ago. Adequate practical arrangements for your sister-in-law's funeral were made. You supported your husband during this process and were 'strong for him'. However, on returning home last week, you feel as if 'things have caught up' with you. You feel physically and mentally drained, but find it difficult to fall asleep and stay asleep. You have tried hot milk with ginger at bedtime to help you sleep but this has not been helpful.

You present to the doctor expecting to discuss how you feel and see if you can get a 'tonic' to help you sleep and feel better.

Information to reveal if asked

General information about yourself:

- Your sister-in-law's death also coincides with the anniversary of a miscarriage. You grieve both losses.

- You are well physically.

- You do not have a past history of anxiety or depression.

- Most of the family are in India. Your children live away from home. You have a small network of friends, mainly work colleagues, with whom you occasionally socialise, either by eating out or going to the cinema.

- You do not smoke and drink wine or gin and tonic only when you eat out.

Further details about your condition:

- You feel tired and fatigued. You have headaches and interrupted sleep. You have difficulty concentrating on your work.

- You are very weepy and irritable. Little incidents, such as your co-worker forgetting to pass on a message, anger you disproportionately. Later on, you feel guilty for your excessive emotional response.

- If specifically asked about the blood tests, you say that you are needle-phobic and have avoided this procedure, as you feel unable to cope with the venepuncture at present. You usually overcome your dread of needles by sheer concentration and willpower.

Your ideas:

- You think that you have bottled up your feelings and you have not dealt with the grief. You think of yourself as stressed and run down, hence your thoughts that a 'tonic' such as St John's wort may help perk you up.

- You have read some spiritual books that advise meditation, but you can't concentrate enough to meditate at present. You are too restless and 'all over the place'.

- If the doctor mentions prescribing tablets, you'd like to know about possible side-effects.

- If the doctor reminds you about your blood test, you ask if you could get a repeat script for the atorvastatin but do the blood test in a few months, when you feel strong enough to cope with your needle phobia.

Your concerns:

- You are worried about not being strong and burdening your husband with your feelings; he lost his only sister and had to help with the complicated and expensive funeral arrangements.

- If you carry on as you are, you may upset colleagues at work and worsen the situation. You worry that things are spiralling out of control but seem powerless to do anything to halt the spiral. You feel hopeless and guilty.

Your expectations:

- You do not expect time off work; you believe it is important to maintain a routine.

- However, it takes a lot more concentration to do the work and you are tired. You would like to feel less tired and ask if taking St John's wort or other tablets may help. You prefer alternative medicines.

Medical history

You are usually healthy and take the atorvastatin for your high cholesterol. You do light exercise and housework. Unfortunately, you have a sweet tooth and have a tendency to indulge in sugary food when stressed.

Social history

You are happily married and your two adult children live away from home.

You enjoy your current social life. You have lived away from the supportive network of a large family for most of your adult life and rarely feel homesick.

Information to reveal if examined

If the doctor asks about depression and anxiety, you feel sad, a bit worried and tired. Your appetite has not really changed; you want to eat sugar probably to help your tiredness. Your weight has not really changed. Your movements are not particularly agitated. You have no thoughts of self-harm.

SUGGESTED APPROACH TO THE CONSULTATION

Targeted history taking:

- What are Aisha's current symptoms? You could subdivide these into 'when you think about your sister-in-law's death, what are the thoughts or images going through your mind? What do you feel when you think these thoughts or see these images? When you think and feel like this, what do you do?'

- What does she think are causing these symptoms?

- Could there be other reasons for these symptoms?

- What treatments has she tried already?

- How are her symptoms affecting her home and work life?

- What are her expectations of this consultation: time off work, medication, advice, or signposting to mental health resources?

- What is her general health like – when is she intending to have her blood tests for cholesterol and liver function?

Targeted examination:

- A brief mental state examination may be all that is required.

- If appropriate, assess suicide risk.

Clinical management:

- Discuss the natural history of a grief reaction. People may experience physical symptoms such as fatigue and headaches as well as psychological symptoms such as 'shock', that is, feelings of unreality, detachment, disbelief or 'numbness'.

- As this is a normal grief reaction rather than a presentation of anxiety, depression, or abnormal grief (such as inhibited, delayed or prolonged grief), an explanation of the 'normality' of the above symptoms may be reassuring.

- Address the patient's ideas: she believes that she needs a tonic for the tiredness. Discuss ways in which tiredness can be improved, such as improving sleep, getting practical help with difficult chores, exercising, taking time out for self, and/or maintaining a routine that includes some enjoyable activities. Some patients find a Cognitive Behaviour Therapy (CBT) framework useful: if you challenge the negative thoughts (*"Talking to my husband will make him feel worse"*) and modify the behaviour (keep to a routine, do things that allow you to experience joy and hope such as meeting friends), then the feelings change (from sadness, hopelessness or anger to optimism, feeling supported or nurtured).

- Address the patient's concerns: she is concerned about burdening her husband by discussing her feelings with him. Explore whether this concern is well founded and whether being more open with him could result in mutual support. Talking about the bereavement can often help to resolve the feelings. The amount of time and discussion needed for people to grieve varies according to the individual.

- Address the patient's expectations: she believes that St John's wort may help with tiredness. St John's wort could be useful. However, St John's wort is known to interfere with many medications, including simvastatin. It may interact with atorvastatin – does she want to consider this option or other measures in the first instance? Negotiate a management plan. Consider prescribing sedatives (zopiclone or diazepam) for a few days.

- Discuss the needle phobia. Consider whether using a topical anaesthetic application or distraction techniques, such as breathing exercises, counting backwards from 300, or listening to music while having blood taken, may be useful.

- Briefly, discuss the importance of cholesterol review and the need to reduce total cholesterol to <5mmol, or preferable <4mmol. Arrange follow-up with results of the blood tests to discuss lifestyle measures and perhaps an increase in the dose of atorvastatin.

- Safety-net: outline when and why follow-up should be arranged for the grief reaction, needle phobia and cholesterol management.

Interpersonal skills:

This case tests how skilfully doctors explore an emotional problem and in particular tests generic GP communication skills: empathy, thoughtful questioning, insightful reflections and positive regard.

A good communicator elicits social information that contextualises the patient's problem, that is, obtains the information about not wanting to burden her husband with her emotional distress. By exploring pros and cons of open discussion with her husband, the doctor and patient may be able to work in partnership to develop a shared management plan.

The treatment involved here includes 'the doctor as a drug'[1], where the rapport and openness of the doctor encourage the patient to unburden her distress, an act that could be therapeutic in itself.

The doctor could also employ some CBT or Motivational Interviewing-type communication skills to allow the patient to make sense of her situation (helping her analyse her thoughts, feelings and behaviours), help her to identify small changes she could make and motivate her to put these plans into action. Such discussion, in contrast to drug prescription alone, empowers the patient and encourages self-sufficiency.

Following the discussion, the doctor could ask, *"What do you think of the discussion we had today? Have you thought of any other suggestions we have not mentioned?".* This may strengthen the therapeutic alliance. To develop an effective alliance, the doctor needs to treat patients as he or she would like to be treated. What the doctor does and says needs to convey their caring and understanding of what the patient is experiencing and their intention to help.

Good communication with the patient explores:

- her agenda (to improve her tiredness and to feel more in control)
- health beliefs (St John's wort and alternative medications are useful remedies) and
- preferences (to delay venepuncture until she is better able to cope with the procedure).

The excellent candidate displays advanced CBT or motivational interviewing skills, such as cost–benefit analysis, motivational scales and problem solving.

Aisha could list the pros and cons of the issue on a piece of paper[2]. On one side of the sheet, she could reflect on the pros of maintaining the status quo, all the reasons for keeping silent to her husband. She also writes down the disadvantages of the proposed new behaviour, in other words all the disadvantages involved in speaking to her husband. On the other side of the paper she writes down the advantages of new behaviour (speaking to husband) and the disadvantages of the status quo (keeping silent). Before embarking on this exercise, it is important to clarify whether the patient is willing to change. If they are fixed in their view that they are right and there is no need to change, there is little point in continuing with the exercise. If they are open to change, they are encouraged to spend time and effort in completing the form for the doctor to review. The doctor reads through the list and asks the patient how committed they are to changing to the new behaviour on a scale of 0 to 10, to come to a greater understanding of their level of motivation. It is important to ask why the motivation is not ranked as zero. This encourages patients to tap into their motives and determination. The doctor asks the patient how they could increase their motivation to 10. This may encourage them to explore certain beliefs they hold about themselves that may be limiting their growth and development. For example, Aisha may say *"My husband works so hard and relaxes in front of the TV. I don't feel it's right to disturb his relaxation".* These beliefs about her perceived powerlessness need to be uncovered and resolved before changes in her thinking can lead to commitment and follow-through. Problem solving techniques are then applied[3].

References

1. Balint, M (2000) *The Doctor, his Patient and the Illness*, 2nd edition. Churchill Livingstone.

2. http://www.montrealcbtpsychologist.com/userfiles/373150/file/Cost_Benefit_Analysis_Worksheet.pdf

3. http://downloads.bbc.co.uk/headroom/cbt/structured_problem_solving.pdf

Relevant literature

Parkes, CM (1998) **Coping with loss: Bereavement in adult life**. *BMJ*, **316(7134)**: 856–859.

A GP visit to the family home on the day after a death can give emotional support to the family. The bereaved may need reassurance that they are not going mad if they break down, that the symptoms of anxiety and tension are not signs of illness, and that it is OK for them to withdraw, for a while, from their accustomed tasks.

As time passes people may also need permission to take a break from grieving – to return to work or do other things that enable them to escape, even briefly, from grief.

The first anniversary is often a time of renewed grieving.

Charlton, R and Dolman, E (1995) **Bereavement: a protocol for primary care**. *Br. J. Gen. Pract.* **45(397)**: 427–430.

Bereavement becomes a medical problem when the surviving intimates become ill. This paper proposes a bereavement protocol to minimize the effects of bereavement.

For information on bereavement, see www.rcpsych.ac.uk/mentalhealthinformation/mentalhealthproblems/bereavement/bereavement.aspx

For information on complementary therapies, see www.rcpsych.ac.uk/mentalhealthinformation/therapies/complementarytherapy.aspx

For communication video-clips, see www.tneel.uic.edu/tneel-ss/demo/connect/frame1.asp

CASE 26 OCD

INFORMATION FOR THE DOCTOR

Name	Aneta Jesien
Age	34
Social and family history	Married, three children
Past medical history	Obsessive Compulsive Disorder (OCD) during last pregnancy 2 years ago
Current medication	Microgynon ED, take 1T daily
Blood tests	Blood tests done antenatally – no problems

INFORMATION FOR THE PATIENT

You are Aneta Jesien, a 34-year-old stay at home mum, who has come to discuss your current emotional distress, your OCD having recurred. You have been fine for eighteen months, since the birth of your baby. During your pregnancy, you developed a fear of catching illnesses, such as toxoplasmosis, which you worried would harm the developing baby. You washed the household surfaces and your hands several times each day. After being diagnosed as having OCD, you saw a psychologist for talking therapies, having declined medication during pregnancy. The talking therapies were very helpful. You felt absolutely fine since the birth of your baby; the fear of catching an illness that would hurt the baby vanished after he was born. Now, you are anxious about driving.

You are deeply afraid of driving. You have to drive the two older children to and from school each day. Your husband can't take them because he commutes and leaves home too early. As school time approaches, you feel yourself getting more anxious and fearful. By the time you leave home, you are in a state of dread. You worry about hitting cyclists and pedestrians. You know this is a 'silly' worry but because you cannot shake it out of your mind, no matter what you do. You think this is a recurrence of your OCD.

You present to the doctor to discuss restarting treatment for your OCD. You feel you cannot go on like this.

Information to reveal if asked

General information about yourself:

- You avoid driving whenever possible. You talk on the phone to your sister and mum in Poland. They are supportive.

- Your husband is understanding of your OCD and reassures you that you are not 'going mad'.

- You are a housewife.

- You are a non-smoker and you do not drink alcohol.

Further details about your condition:

- When your husband went away on business three weeks ago, you had to look after your three boys on your own. You had to do more driving during this period. The symptoms started at this point. You have been driving for more than ten years and have never had any accidents or convictions.

- You worry whether your car is passing too close to cyclists and pedestrians and whether you would know if you injured them. You see images of the injured people in your mind.

- When you drive, your palms are sweaty. You feel tense and fearful. You feel angry with yourself for allowing these silly fears to take root. You feel exhausted from controlling the urge to go back along the route to check for injured people.

- If specifically asked, the fear of driving now dominates a large part of your morning and afternoon. Once you return home, you force yourself to not go back along the route to check for accident victims. You distract yourself by getting on with the housework and playing with the baby, but the images of accident victims keep popping into your mind. You feel exhausted and agitated.

Your ideas:

- You think that your OCD has recurred.

- You tried re-reading your book, *Overcoming Anxiety*, which you found very useful during your pregnancy. It does not seem to help any more. You have tried the relaxation and breathing techniques the psychologist previously advised. These helped to calm you but did not make the fear of driving disappear.

- If the doctor suggests prescribing tablets, you'd like to know about possible side-effects.

- If the doctor offers a referral, you indicate that you do not want a referral to community mental health (CMH) because you associate seeing the psychologists with the way you felt during your pregnancy.

Your concerns:

- You are worried about 'taking out' your feelings on your children. You are quite curt with the children on the drive to school because their noise may distract you. You feel guilty for treating them in this way.

- You are worried about the OCD having come back. You had hoped that everything went away after you gave birth.

Your expectations:

- You think the doctor will refer you to CMH but this means you will have to drive to the town centre. There are no quiet back roads to their offices. There isn't a convenient bus service. You would prefer to be treated at the GP surgery.

Medical history

You are usually healthy.

Social history

You are happily married, but your husband's job often takes him away from home for several days at a time. Your 3 boys are all under 8, and though well-behaved, can be a handful. You have a supportive network of friends.

Information to reveal if examined

If the doctor asks about depression and anxiety, you do not feel sad but you do feel anxious, ranging from mild worry to almost full-blown panic depending on the situation. Your stomach gets tied into knots and you don't want to eat. Your weight has not really changed. You have no thoughts of self-harm. You sleep from 9.30pm to 6am. You do not wake during the night. You do not feel uninterested in things.

SUGGESTED APPROACH TO THE CONSULTATION

Targeted history taking:

- What are her current symptoms?

- Elicit the thoughts that are making her anxious, that is, her obsessions.

- Elicit the way in which her anxiety manifests itself, such as her feelings and/or physical symptoms of anxiety such as headaches, palpitations and chest pain.

- Elicit the things she does to reduce the anxiety, that is, her compulsive behaviours.

- Has anything happened recently that could have provoked the anxiety, such as stress or life changes?

- How are her symptoms affecting her home and work life?

- Is there any associated co-morbidity such as depression?

- What treatments has she already tried?

- What are her expectations of this consultation: signposting to self-help information, referral to mental health services or initiation of medication?

- What is her general health like – how much is she smoking or drinking?

Targeted examination:

- A brief mental state examination may be required.

- If she is washing her hands recurrently, briefly examine for dry or fissured skin.

Clinical management:

- Based on her symptoms, it looks like Aneta is correct in her diagnosis that her OCD has relapsed. It may help to discuss the natural history and possible aetiology of OCD.

- Reassure her that her husband is correct in saying that people with OCD are not 'mad'; help to de-stigmatise mental illness.

- Congratulate her on not getting into the ritual of checking for accident victims. Rituals may briefly reduce anxiety; however, they strengthen the belief that fixed patterns of behaviour can stop negative things from happening.

- Address the patient's ideas: she believes that seeing a psychologist will trigger the feelings she had during her pregnancy. It may be appropriate to explore this in greater detail and find out her reasons, experiences and emotions regarding the CMH psychology services. To balance this negative perspective, the doctor may want to discover how previous contact was useful. Ask Aneta if she can think of anything to reduce her fear of contacting the mental health services; for example, would seeing them at an alternative venue be less stressful?

- Address Aneta's concerns about the effect the OCD is having on her relationship with her children. She may need to be reminded that OCD is treatable and that she regained control of her feelings and behaviour in the past; encourage optimism and hope.

- Address Aneta's expectations: she would like treatment in Primary Care. Discuss possible options: referral to the practice counsellor for exposure and response prevention or cognitive therapy; or guided self-help using books such as *Overcoming Obsessive-Compulsive Disorder: a self-help book using cognitive-behavioural techniques* by David Veale and Rob Willson; or treatment with SSRIs to reduce obsessions and compulsions. Negotiate a management plan. If you prescribe medication, take steps to encourage concordance.

- Safety-net: outline when and why you would next like to see Aneta. If you refer Aneta, discuss when she is likely to hear from the team and what she should do if she has not heard from anyone within a specified period.

Interpersonal skills:

In this case the patient knows and understands her diagnosis, which after taking a history, the doctor confirms. There is no diagnostic dilemma. What the case does test is the doctor's ability to negotiate the treatment plan with the patient. Negotiation involves an array of communication skills to resolve conflict.

Conflict may arise in this case because what the patient and doctor want differ. The patient wants to avoid driving to CMH. The doctor may want the patient to engage with CMH, a previously successful treatment and to challenge her fear of driving. It could become so easy, if Aneta stopped driving, for her to become isolated. Both sides have to discuss their views and emotions and acknowledge the other's position. Both parties need to come up with proposals and options for discussion and consideration before settling on the mutually accepted solution. The steps going forward need to be clarified.

The good communicator displays several negotiation skills, namely active listening and asking questions to clarify the situation to gain a better understanding of what is happening. Tolerance, acceptance, and being non-judgemental are important attributes. The sensitive GP accepts that people are different, with differing abilities and strengths. Hence, they adjust their communication to the person sitting in front of them so that their messages are clear, simple and succinct.

Poor communication with the patient:

- fails to elicit a thorough history of her thoughts (obsessions), feelings (anxiety/dread) and behaviours (avoidance behaviour, constantly seeking reassurance).

- fails to explore how the patient's life is affected by the problem – how a large portion of the day is spent thinking about accident victims and how the emotional burden is fatiguing her.

- fails to encourage self-sufficiency – referral to the mental health team or psychologist without exploration of her fears, and without offering self-help measures can be perceived as instructing the patient rather than adopting an approach that is responsive to the patient's preferences, feelings and expectations.

Therefore, poor communicators show little understanding of their patients' illness and its psychosocial impact. Consequently, their management plan contains a number of instructions, most of which fail to empower the patient and nurture self-sufficiency.

Additional reading

Heyman, I et al. (2006) **Obsessive-compulsive disorder**. BMJ, **333**: 424–429.

- Obsessions are intrusive thoughts (ideas, images, or impulses) that repeatedly enter a person's mind against his or her will, generating considerable anxiety.
- Compulsions are repetitive acts – attempts or rituals to reduce the anxiety caused by the obsessions, but the relief is only temporary.
- With time, 'automatic' rituals can increase, rather than reduce, the anxiety.
- Ritualising may maintain the problem – the patient fails to deal with their fears and their anxiety.
- The aim of exposure and response prevention, a psychological therapy, is to break this cycle by persuading patients to expose themselves to the feared situations and, at the same time, to refrain from performing any rituals.

Relevant literature

For a patient leaflet on OCD, see:

www.rcpsych.ac.uk/mentalhealthinformation/mentalhealthproblems/obsessivecompulsivedisorder/obsessivecomplusivedisorder.aspx

For NICE (2005) guidance on OCD management, including treatment in primary care, see: www.nice.org.uk/guidance/cg31

University of Kent Persuading, Influencing and Negotiating Skills www.kent.ac.uk/careers/sk/persuading.htm

CASE 27 Confidentiality

INFORMATION FOR THE DOCTOR

You are a doctor in surgery. You are visited by DC Peter Kerr, Criminal Investigations Department, requesting more information about your patient Robert Smith in relation to an alleged assault.

Name	Robert Smith
Age	34
Social and family history	<ul><li>Unemployed</li><li>Smoker: 20 cigarettes/day</li><li>Alcohol: 30–35 units/week</li><li>Ex-heroin user</li></ul>
Medical history	<ul><li>Borderline personality disorder</li><li>IV drug user (heroin) 15 years ago</li><li>Methadone programme 12 years ago</li><li>Alcohol abuse: attempted detox programme 10 years ago – failed</li><li>Hepatitis B positive 12 years ago, no record since then about the condition</li><li>Several A&E attendances for alcohol related incidents in last 10 years (involving minor injury/burns, etc.)</li><li>Anger management programme 2 years ago</li></ul>

The medical record of his **last consultation** 1 week ago reads:

"Gastritis – related to binge drinking with friends over the weekend. Prescribed omeprazole 20mg for 28 days. Admits to being clean (no illicit drugs for last 13 years). Not interested in referral to 'alcohol detoxification' programmes."

INFORMATION FOR THE PATIENT

This is a third party consultation. You are Detective Constable Peter Kerr, Criminal Investigations Department. You are here to obtain more information on Mr Robert Smith.

You are investigating Mr Smith for an assault on his partner Ms Vera Moore.

Your opening statement is *"Good morning Doctor, I am DC Peter Kerr. This is about your patient Robert Smith; we are investigating him for assault and damage to property."*

You have the following information about patient Robert Smith:

Robert has been living with his partner Ms Vera Moore, aged 24. She works at a bar. He was involved in an altercation with Ms Moore two days ago. The situation got out of hand and Robert assaulted Vera. She was punched in the face and kicked in the abdomen and chest. She has sustained a broken nose and fractured ribs. She has been discharged from A&E and is stable.

Ms Moore is not a patient in your surgery; she has reported the incident to the police and they have her consent to discuss matters for this investigation.

Information to reveal if asked

General information about Robert Smith:

- You know from Vera and from your police records that Robert is an ex-heroin addict and has a criminal record for assault and burglary 7 years ago. He served a jail sentence of 6 months for that burglary. Since his release from prison, he has managed to stay out of trouble.

Further details about current incident:

- You are concerned about Robert's drinking and its implications for his family's safety. There is a particular concern about Vera's children (3-year-old daughter and 5-year-old son from previous relationship). Currently the children are with their grandmother (Vera's mother).

- The children are on the child protection register (due to previous NAI where the 3-year-old daughter had sustained unexplained bruises. This was fully investigated 2 years ago and except for Robert and Vera not being charged, you are unaware of any other outcomes).

- The children were not involved this time and are unharmed.

Your ideas:

- You know Robert is binge drinking. This information was provided by Vera.
- The police found empty beer cans and vodka bottles in his flat. Robert was completely drunk at the time of the incident. You think it is his excessive alcohol and possible drugs which is causing disharmony in the couple's relationship.

Your concerns:

- You are worried about alcohol and drug use, and their potential impact on Vera's young children, who live with the couple.
- You will be contacting Vera's GP for more information on her children.
- Robert has forensic history, has been involved in assault. There was knife use during one of his burglaries 7 years ago.

Your expectations:

- You want to know if Robert is on any illicit drugs. Is he currently on an alcohol- or drug-related programme? How much is he drinking? Is he at risk of binge drinking and alcohol-fuelled impulsive behaviour?
- As his GP, do you have any other relevant information?

SUGGESTED APPROACH TO THE CONSULTATION

Targeted history taking:

- Take a detailed history of the incident. In particular, you need to assess the risk to Vera and her children from Robert's current alcohol consumption and mental state.

Targeted examination:

- Not needed in this case; this is a third party consultation.

Clinical management:

- Carry out a risk assessment – what is the risk to Vera and her young children from domestic violence? The children are with their grandmother, so not in imminent danger. But when are they due to return home? Where is Robert? Where is Vera? How is Vera being kept safe?

- The police do not have the authority to demand a disclosure of patient information or patient identifiable information. However, there are certain situations where a doctor is required to provide the police with information, with or without patient consent. This is especially important in situations when the doctor is acting in the public interest; where there is significant danger to other individuals or the public at large. Therefore, in this case, it is important to consider the benefit of passing on to the police information that may be relevant:
  - Robert is currently binge drinking and may act impulsively when drunk;
  - he has borderline personality disorder (old records may give information about whether he has difficulty controlling his emotions and thoughts, examples of impulsive behaviour and whether he has a history of unstable relationships);
  - recent examination did not comment on objective evidence of drug use – there is no documentation of injection sites being seen/infected;
  - he recently declined referral to an alcohol detox programme.

- After weighing up the risk and benefit of passing on some or none of the above information, obtain further information from DC Kerr. What do the police know or suspect about possible drug use? How dangerous do they suspect him of being and what information do they base this assessment on?

- Consider your options: taking DC Kerr's details, discussing the case with the MDU, checking with patient that he understands that his GP has been contacted by the police and finding out whether he is OK with certain information being passed to them. Consider whether the doctor–patient trust may encourage him to present in surgery and ask for help with his alcohol problem. It sounds like he has hit rock bottom and may be in need of support and medical help.

BACKGROUND KNOWLEDGE REQUIRED FOR THIS CASE

GMC guidance – Justifiable disclosures in the public interest

"The disclosure of information about a patient without their express consent may be justifiable, if the public interest in disclosing the information outweighs the patient's interests in keeping it confidential.

In all cases, you must decide whether or not the possible harm caused to the patient – and the overall trust between doctors and patients – by disclosing this information will outweigh the benefits resulting from the disclosure.

You should try to ensure that the information is anonymised, if practicable, and that you are only disclosing information relevant to the purpose of the disclosure. Only in exceptional circumstances should non-anonymised data be disclosed.

You should attempt to seek the patient's consent, but there are certain circumstances when this will not be possible – for example, if the patient lacks capacity, you are not able to trace the patient, obtaining consent undermines the purposes for which the disclosure was being made, or the disclosure must be made quickly, such as cases of detection or control of communicable diseases.

It is important to document any decision you make and your reasons for disclosing the information."

Legal obligations to disclose information (from GMC guidance)

1. Court orders – when doctor is presented with a court order for disclosure of information, he must disclose information. (In complex situations seek advice from defence union/Caldicott guardian/hospital solicitors.)
2. Evidence of serious crime
3. Gunshot wounds
4. Knife wounds
5. Domestic abuse and children, sexual abuse and rape
6. Abuse/neglect victims who lack capacity to consent disclosure.

This is a very tricky case. The aim of the case is to see if the doctor can weigh up risk/benefit to patient vs. risk/benefit to Vera/children/society. The doctor has to balance a duty of care to their patient with a duty of care to the public. To score well, you must be able to gather data to inform your risk management. You must also discuss the risks and benefits of disclosing confidential information (in general terms to DC Kerr) so that he understands why you are proceeding with caution and does not label you as being obstructive. You need to end the discussion with a plan: either disclose information, justifying why you are doing so; or agree to speak to DC Kerr later, but inform him of your intention to speak to the patient and MDU first. You should give DC Kerr realistic time lines.

In this case, a doctor may be justified in giving information about the patient's alcohol/drug use or recent attendance for binge drinking, without his consent. Two minor children are involved and their safety is paramount.

Relevant literature

Department of Health (1997) *The Caldicott Committee Report on the Review of Patient-Identifiable Information.* www.wales.nhs.uk/sites3/Documents/950/DH_4068404.pdf

GMC (2009) *Confidentiality.* www.gmc-uk.org/guidance/ethical_guidance/confidentiality.asp

CASE 28 Emergency contraception

INFORMATION FOR THE DOCTOR

Name	Nicole Hess
Age	19
Social and family history	• Married, works as a shop assistant • Non-smoker, alcohol 6 units/week
Past medical history	None

INFORMATION FOR THE PATIENT

You are Nicole Hess, a 19-year-old assistant in a perfume shop. You are recently married. You live with your husband. He works in a supermarket and is 26 years old. You do not have children and no plans for a pregnancy for a couple of years.

You are here for emergency contraception. Your opening statement is *"Good morning Doctor, can I have the morning after pill?"*.

Information to reveal if asked

General information about yourself:

- You finished school after GCSEs and have done odd jobs. You have worked in cosmetic shops and enjoyed working in the beauty sections. You are currently working at the Dior counter in a high street shop.

- You have known your husband for two years; you married eight months ago. You are not ready for children yet as both are struggling financially and have a debt of £10,000. You live in a rented flat in an expensive part of the city and have high outgoings.

- Your husband is a graphic designer, is still paying off his student loan and is looking for jobs. He took up the supermarket job as it is close to your flat and will help in paying off some bills.

Further details about your condition:

- You have regular 28-day cycles and bleed for 5 days. You usually use condoms. You are not on regular contraception. You tried the pill 3 years ago but it affected your mood and you believe it made you put on some weight. You haven't been on hormonal contraception since.

- You had unprotected sex a week ago. You had your LMP 3 weeks ago.

- You used the morning after pill last year. You are not aware of the time frames.

Your ideas:

- You think the morning after pill works any time before your next period. Your period is due in a week. If you fall pregnant, then you will have to think about it. You are not sure if you can go ahead with a pregnancy and are worried about the possibility of getting pregnant.

- You are not keen on an IUD.

Your concerns:

- You are worried that you might get pregnant if the morning after pill fails.

- Your main concern about a possible pregnancy is that the child may not belong to your husband. You have had a fling with your colleague at work and you did not use condoms. You came to the GP late as you had not had time to do so before. You do not want to go ahead with the pregnancy if the baby is not your husband's. You want to know about paternity tests and your colleague is willing to give a blood test if needed.

Your expectations:

- You want the morning after pill.
- You want to know what the chances of pill failure are, or of you getting pregnant.
- If you do fall pregnant you would like to have a paternity test before making a decision to continue with the pregnancy.

SUGGESTED APPROACH TO THE CONSULTATION

Targeted history taking:
- Obtain details of patient's menstrual cycle and time of unprotected sex.
- Find out about any medications or use of contraceptive methods.
- Get a detailed sexual history including number of partners or sexual activity.

Targeted examination:
- No medical examination needed.

Clinical management:
- Clarify patient's concepts about emergency contraception use.
- Discuss time frames regarding different emergency contraceptive methods and inform patient that she is too late for most methods.
- Discuss the need for STI check and follow-up.
- Discuss the need for pregnancy test if her period is late.
- Arrange a follow-up appointment and provide information on paternity tests, which are not available on NHS.

Interpersonal skills:
Good communication with the patient:
- Is non-judgemental regarding her sexual encounter.
- Offers information in a manner she understands and addresses concerns about the possible pregnancy.
- Offers a follow-up plan.

BACKGROUND KNOWLEDGE REQUIRED FOR THIS CASE

Types of emergency contraception available:
Levonelle (pill) should be taken within three days (72 hours) of unprotected sex. It can be used from day 21 of giving birth or after a miscarriage or abortion.

EllaOne (pill) can be taken within five days (120 hours) of unprotected sex.

Avoid breastfeeding for 36 hours after taking EllaOne.

Emergency IUD can be fitted up to 5 days after unprotected sex.

Paternity testing:
Paternity testing is not available on the NHS and patients may have to pay for it privately.

Samples are needed:

Blood from pregnant woman, amniocentesis or chorionic villus sampling.

Blood sample or cheek cells from male partner are needed.

Under the Human Tissue Act 2004, prenatal paternity tests done in the UK must have the consent of the man involved.

Relevant literature

FPA (www.fpa.org.uk/contraception-help/emergency-contraception)

NHS Choices (www.nhs.uk/chq/pages/what-is-a-prenatal-paternity-test.aspx)

CASE 29 Hirsutism

INFORMATION FOR THE DOCTOR

Name	Agata Kwiatkowski
Age	26
Social and family history	Single
Past medical history	None

INFORMATION FOR THE PATIENT

You are Agata Kwiatkowski, a 26-year-old single woman, with signs of hirsutism.

You are very embarrassed about your excessive hair which you think has worsened over the last three years. You thread and pluck out the hair but have never tried any medical treatment for it. You started working in a hotel spa three years ago and have been busy, with no time for exercise. You think you have gained substantial weight over the three years as a result of binge eating; you enjoy the desserts and sweets at this expensive hotel which are available free of charge.

You are currently single, having recently broken up with your boyfriend of two years. You sometimes think that it is your 'manly appearance' which triggered the breakdown in the relationship.

Your opening statement is *"Doctor, I've got this embarrassing problem. I have excessive hair on my chest and chin"*.

Information to reveal if asked
General information about yourself:

- You broke up with your boyfriend because he cheated on you with a friend who is slimmer and prettier.

- You think that your excessive hair is a turn-off for men.

- You have gained 2 stone in weight in the last 3 years.

- You have been working in health- and beauty-related professions for the last 7 years. You have worked in beauty salons and massage parlours prior to your current job.

- You had dated few men and this was your first serious relationship. You were with your Italian boyfriend for 2 years before the breakup.

Medical history

- Previously you were fit and well with no medical problems.

- Menstrual history: menarche at 14 years. Your cycles were always irregular but have got worse lately. You have scanty painless bleeds for 2–3 days and cycles can vary from 45 days to 3 months.

- There is no history of constipation or cold intolerance. There is no change in bowel habit or voice, nor are there any skin changes. You always had excessive facial and chest hair since your teenage years. The weight gain has been progressive since you took up the new job.

Social history

You live alone, do not smoke and drink 10 units of alcohol per week.

Information to reveal if examined

If the doctor asks to weigh you, hand him/her a card saying "BMI 30".

BP 122/73mmHg

Abdominal examination normal

SUGGESTED APPROACH TO THE CONSULTATION

Targeted history taking:

- Does excessive hair growth run in her family?
- Pattern of hirsutism in relation to puberty, details of her menstrual history and any related problems.
- Any changes in her weight or any recent weight gain, pattern of obesity; truncal obesity?
- Any features which could suggest an increase in androgens such as thinning of scalp hair, deepening of voice, acne, increased libido, loss of breast tissue?
- Has she commenced on any new medications recently?
- What symptoms are causing the greatest distress?
- Has she considered other therapies for excessive hair growth like electrolysis and laser therapy, waxing or shaving?

Targeted examination:

- Perform a physical examination; important aspects are weight and BMI.
- Take BP and carry out an abdominal examination.

Clinical management:

- Address patient's concerns and issues about her weight gain.
- First line management to include advice on lifestyle changes to reduce weight: diet, exercise.
- Offer baseline blood tests: testosterone, TSH, glucose (random or fasting) or HbA1c.
- Discuss options to induce a menstrual bleed. A BMI of 30 puts her in a UKMEC category of 2 with regard to the CHC. Discuss the risks and benefits of CHC so the patient can make an informed choice.
- Discuss options of eflornithine cream for facial hair.
- Discuss options of topical cosmetic therapies for hair reduction and removal.

Interpersonal skills:

Good communication with the patient:

- explores her agenda (to reduce the hirsutism)
- discovers her health beliefs (would reducing her weight help?)
- finds out her preferences.

This can then result in an agreed management plan.

BACKGROUND KNOWLEDGE REQUIRED FOR THIS CASE

The Rotterdam 2003 Criteria for defining PCOS, after exclusion of related disorders, involve finding two of the following three features:

1. Clinical oligomenorrhoea or amenorrhoea; cycles more than 35 days or less than 10 periods a year
2. Clinical or biochemical evidence of hyperandrogenism (hirsutism, acne, alopecia or raised free androgen index)
3. Polycystic ovaries on USS.

NICE Hirsutism summary (CKS December 2013)

http://cks.nice.org.uk/hirsutism#!topicsummary

Hirsutism is growth of excess terminal hair on the face, chest, linea alba, lower back, buttocks and anterior thighs in women.

In premenopausal women PCOS is the most common cause of hirsutism (>70% of cases). No apparent underlying cause is found in about quarter of women. Androgen-secreting tumours, congenital adrenal hyperplasia, Cushing's syndrome, acromegaly and drugs are less common causes.

Management options in primary care:

- Weight loss if obese or overweight
- Hair reduction and removal treatments
- Eflornithine cream (for facial hirsutism in women aged 19 years or older)
- A combined COC, provided there are no contraindications. Options are Dianette (co-cyprindiol, licensed use) or a COC containing drospirenone (e.g. Yasmin, unlicensed use).

Referral to a specialist is recommended if:

- there are clinical features suggestive of an androgen-secreting tumour
- there are clinical features of Cushing's syndrome
- hair growth worsens despite treatment
- treatment has not been effective after at least 6 months.

NICE Polycystic ovary syndrome (CKS 2013)

http://cks.nice.org.uk/polycystic-ovary-syndrome

Overview of management:

- Encourage a healthy lifestyle to reduce possible long-term risks to health (type 2 diabetes and cardiovascular disease).
- Do not initiate treatment with insulin-sensitising drugs (metformin) in primary care. Refer women if this treatment is considered.

- Offer regular screening for cardiovascular risk factors, specifically impaired glucose tolerance and type 2 diabetes.
- Ask about snoring and daytime fatigue/somnolence.
- For women with oligomenorrhoea or amenorrhoea: Induce a withdrawal bleed and then refer for ultrasonography to assess endometrial thickness. If endometrium fails to shed or has unusual appearance, refer to exclude endometrial hyperplasia or cancer.

CASE 30 Viral infection

INFORMATION FOR THE DOCTOR

You are a doctor in surgery. You receive a phone call from Chloe Novak, who wishes to discuss how her son Jack's childhood illness may affect her pregnancy.

Name	Mrs Chloe Novak
Age	26
Social and family history	• Married • Health care assistant, works in A&E department • Non-smoker, alcohol 4 units/week

INFORMATION FOR THE PATIENT

You are Chloe Novak, 26 years old. You are married, live with your husband in a semi-detached house. You have a 6-year-old son. You work as a health care assistant in the local A&E. You work part-time, three days a week.

You have rung the doctor for advice on your son's health. He has had a flu-like illness and been off school for two days.

Information to reveal if asked

Details about your son's condition:

- You want advice about your 6-year-old son Jack Novak. He has been unwell for a few days. He started with a 'flu-like illness' a week ago, complained about vague aches and pains and today has come up in a rash.

- He does not have a temperature (done on a home thermometer). He has stayed off school and seems well in himself. He is playing about, eating and drinking as usual. There is no vomiting or diarrhoea, he does not complain of headaches or neck pain or light hurting his eyes.

- The rash is on his cheeks and is bright pink. There is no rash on his body. It fades on deep pressure.

- He is otherwise in good health with no symptoms at all.

Your ideas:

- You work in A&E and have seen similar rashes; you think it is 'slapped cheek disease'.

Your concerns:

- You are not worried about Jack, you know this is a viral infection and he will get better in a few days.

- You have some specific concerns. You are 32 weeks pregnant and are concerned if your son's infection will affect the unborn baby.

Your expectations:

- You want advice on the condition.

- You want to know if you need any vaccinations.

Medical history

- You are fit and well, not on any medications.

- Your pregnancy has been uneventful, all scans and checks normal.

- Jack has been a healthy child with no medical problems. All his vaccinations are up to date.

SUGGESTED APPROACH TO THE CONSULTATION

Targeted history taking:

- Take a detailed history of Jack's condition, type of rash; its distribution, duration and progress. Obtain information about the quality of rash if fading on pressure, and use of glass test.

- Get details on his general condition, fever, vomiting, headache or any breathing problems.

- Find out about patient's pregnancy, any other medical conditions and patient's health.

Clinical management:

- Reassure patient regarding Jack and her pregnancy.

- Provide information about parvovirus B19 virus, its implications and associated risks in a manner the patient understands.

- Offer a follow-up for routine review for both mother and child.

BACKGROUND KNOWLEDGE REQUIRED FOR THIS CASE

Current guidelines

- UK antenatal screening programme covers rubella, syphilis, HIV and Hepatitis (NHS screening committee) (www.dh.gov.uk)

Infections in pregnancy

Parvovirus B19

Parvovirus B19 is the cause of fifth disease and slapped cheek disease or erythema infectiosum. Women infected with parvovirus B19 during the first 20 weeks of pregnancy have an increased risk of miscarriage. The risk of an adverse outcome of pregnancy after this is remote.

Women who are infected during weeks 9 to 20 of pregnancy have a low risk (3%) that the baby will develop fetal hydrops.

If parvovirus infection occurs before 20 weeks, it is worthwhile checking parvovirus serology and if positive, ultrasound scans to monitor fetal growth.

Chickenpox

Chickenpox occurs in pregnancy in about 3 per 1000 woman in the UK. About 90% of women have antibodies to varicella zoster virus (VZV) and therefore the fetus is not at risk of chickenpox even when the mother develops shingles during pregnancy. In the non-immune pregnant woman, chickenpox is potentially dangerous, associated with fetal and maternal morbidity and mortality.

Chickenpox infection in pregnant women can lead to varicella pneumonitis. Risk is higher after 20 weeks of gestation, in those who smoke, have chronic lung disease, are immunosuppressed or have more than 100 skin lesions.

Fetal varicella syndrome is a known complication in the first half of pregnancy. Risk is 0.5% of maternal chickenpox in pregnancies of 2–12 weeks; 1.4% between 12 and 28 weeks, and 0% from 20 weeks onwards.

Shingles in a pregnant woman does not pose a risk to infant.

HIV

Up to 50% of infants of HIV-seropositive mothers are pre- or perinatally infected with HIV.

Zidovudine reduces the incidence of vertical transmission of HIV from 26% to 8%. This treatment is effective regardless of the mother's viral load.

Caesarean section may halve the risk relative to normal delivery.

Rubella

Rubella infection during pregnancy is potentially teratogenic and can cause the congenital rubella syndrome.

Risk of fetal infection is greatest if maternal infection occurs during the first trimester.

Fetal damage occurs in up to 90% of cases of maternal rubella infection in first 8–10 weeks. Risk of fetal damage declines to about 10–20% by 16 weeks. Fetal damage as a result of maternal rubella infection is rare after 16 weeks of gestation.

Immunity to rubella is not always lifelong and therefore immunity should be checked at booking. If rubella infection is suspected during pregnancy expert advice should be sought. The diagnosis should always be confirmed via virus isolation or antibody tests showing seroconversion or specific IgM. This is irrespective of history of immunisation, clinical rubella or previous positive rubella antibody test.

Hepatitis B

HBV is transmitted through sexual contact, contaminated blood (e.g. needle sharing) and vertical transmission.

The screening test identifies Hepatitis B surface antigen (HBSAg) and has an accuracy of 99.9%. The presence of Hep B e antigen indicates high infectivity.

DoH states that all pregnant women should be offered screening for Hepatitis B. All babies born to infected mothers should receive a complete course of immunisation starting at birth.

Relevant literature

CDC (1994) **Zidovudine for the prevention of HIV transmission from mother to infant**. *Morb. Mortal. Wkly Rep.* **43**: 285–287.

Drug and Therapeutics Bulletin (2005) **Chickenpox, pregnancy and the newborn**. **43(9)**: 69–72.

The European Collaborative Study (1994) **Caesarian section and risk of vertical transmission of HIV-1 infection**. *Lancet*, **343**: 1464–1467.

GP notebook. **Screening for hepatitis B in pregnancy**. www.gpnotebook.co.uk/simplepage.cfm?ID=x20070130132353295600

The Green Book (1996) **Immunisation against infectious disease**. HMSO.

RCOG (2007) **Chickenpox in pregnancy**.

Miller, W (1998) **Immediate and long term outcome of human parvovirus B19 infection in pregnancy**. *Br. J. Obs. Gyn.* **105**: 174–178.

Tunbridge, AJ *et al.* (2008) **Chickenpox in adults – Clinical management**. *Journal of Infection*, **57**: 95–102.

CASE 31 Abdominal pain

INFORMATION FOR THE DOCTOR

Name	Robert Mitchell
Age	30 years
Social and family history	• Employed as IT consultant • Non-smoker, alcohol 20 units/week
Past medical history	• Tinea pedis • Fracture radius 3 years ago
Current medication	None
Blood tests FBC	*Blood tests done a week ago*
	Hb	13.3g/dL
	WBC	9.5×10^9/L (4.0–10.0)
	Platelets	208×10^9 (150–400)
	Haematocrit	40% (40–53)
	ESR	35mm/h (1–12)
U&Es	Na	140mmol/L (135–145)
	K	3.8mmol/L (3.5–5.5)
	Cl	104mmol/L (90–110)
	Cr	90µmol/L (60–120)
LFTs	Albumin	45 g/L (35–50)
	Bilirubin	12µmol/L (<21)
	ALP	80IU/L (39–150)
	AST	19IU/L (5–40)
	ALT	13IU/L (5–40)

The medical record of his **last consultation** in surgery with your colleague Dr Brown 10 days ago reads:

"Diarrhoea – loose stools about 4 times per day; minor tummy ache; using Imodium OTC. Just returned from New York so possible infection. Recent promotion with increase in work responsibilities so may be IBS. Get bloods and stool culture, then review."

Stool culture negative for *E. coli*/salmonella/shigella/campylobacter.

INFORMATION FOR THE PATIENT

You are Robert Mitchell, a 30-year-old man. You are a highly placed IT consultant at American Express. You have a busy job which involves frequent international travel.

You live in a rented flat with your fiancée. She is 26 years old and has just started working in a law firm. You are in a stable relationship and life is good.

You have been having abdominal pain and loose stools for over 2 months. This is not associated with nausea or vomiting. You have also had mouth ulcers on and off.

A GP colleague had asked for blood tests a week ago. You are here to discuss the blood results and have some medicines.

Information to reveal if asked

General information about yourself:

- You have recently got a promotion and a salary hike. You are now the lead IT consultant in the firm. This brings with it added responsibility and new challenges. You sometimes have work pressures but are enjoying your role.

- You travel frequently for business meetings; you returned from New York 10 days ago and had travelled to Frankfurt a month ago. Your last holiday was in Thailand 6 months ago. This trip was taken with your fiancée. You were fine on the trip and did not have any problems on returning.

- You are in a stable relationship with Emma. You met her at a business meeting and clicked straight away. You have been together for 5 years and are due to get married next week. Emma is Australian; her family lives in Sydney and you are due to fly to Australia in a week's time. Emma has already flown over to Sydney and is busy with the marriage preparations. The family has planned a grand wedding and you are looking forward to it.

Further details about your condition:

- Symptoms have now worsened, with increase in frequency of stools with blood and mucus. You were having some abdominal pain and loose stools for 2 months but have now had bloody diarrhoea for a week.

- You think you have lost some weight. You still have a good appetite but are scared to eat.

- You have had mouth ulcers on and off and have some at the moment.

- You do not have any joint pains, any eye symptoms or skin lesions.

- You are taking Imodium over the counter but it hasn't helped. You have been drinking plenty of water and avoiding alcohol and spicy food which upsets your stomach.

Your ideas:

- You think it could be irritable bowel; one of your cousins has had the condition for years and takes Imodium as needed. You have tried the medication for 2 weeks with no effect. You think you might need antibiotics for a possible tummy bug.

Your concerns:

- Your big day is next Friday and you need to get better to fly and go ahead with the wedding.
- You are worried that this could be IBS which is worsened with a possible stomach bug.

Your expectations:

- You want a stronger drug for symptom relief. You have given a stool sample as recommended by another GP.
- You want antibiotics if the stool sample shows infection.
- You have to get this diarrhoea under control urgently. You are unable to cancel this trip. You are happy to see a consultant privately if necessary as you have health insurance.

Medical history

Previously you were fit and well with no medical problems. You had a fungal infection, if that counts, which was treated with a cream.

Social history

You need to use the toilet 3–4 times daily in the office. Your bowel habits have actually started interfering with your life. You travel a lot for business meetings and work-related issues. Abdominal pain and loose bowels interfere with daily activities.

There have been times where you had to leave business meetings due to abdominal pain.

You are unable to socialise or pursue your hobbies. You don't go to the gym any more as you feel tired by the end of the day. You are concerned about the impact on your life.

Information to reveal if examined

- Abdomen soft, tender left iliac fossa, no masses, PR declined. No guarding/rigidity.
- Temperature 36.2°C.

SUGGESTED APPROACH TO THE CONSULTATION

Targeted history taking:

- Take a detailed history of Robert's diarrhoea; its duration, frequency, associated blood or mucus.
- Are there any red flags like loss of weight (of ≥5%), night diarrhoea, blood in stool and family history of IBD or colon cancer?
- History of travel, any restaurant meals or food-related incidents.
- Family history of any gastrointestinal problems.
- History related to extra-intestinal symptoms.

Targeted examination:

- Examine for signs of iron or vitamin deficiency (stomatitis or glossitis), mouth ulcers, pallor, arthritis, uveitis, abdominal mass or perianal disease.
- Abdominal examination.

Clinical management:

- Discuss patient's concerns and the possible diagnosis of IBD (inflammatory bowel disease). Discuss blood and stool results. Consider requesting a faecal calprotectin blood test.
- Check patient's understanding of proposed diagnosis and clarify his doubts regarding IBS and infective gastroenteritis.
- Take into account patient's circumstances including impending wedding in Australia, and offer support.
- Arrange prompt private referral to gastroenterologist as per patient's wishes, and follow-up. Treatment to be initiated as per local protocols or on (telephone) advice of gastroenterology team while awaiting the appointment. There is usually a shared management plan. Reassure the patient that acute mild to moderate colitis, when treated with a combination of oral and topical mesalazine, usually results in remission for about 60% of patients.

Interpersonal skills:

Good communication with patient:

- Offers information in a way the patient can understand.
- Shows empathy and offers support, taking into account patient's circumstances.
- Works with the patient to agree on a treatment plan or referral.

BACKGROUND KNOWLEDGE REQUIRED FOR THIS CASE

NICE guidelines on Crohn's disease (CG152, October 2012)

Give information, advice and support in line with NICE guidance on smoking cessation, patient experience, medicine adherence, fertility and additional information on following when appropriate:

- Possible delay of growth and puberty in children and young people
- Diet and nutrition
- Fertility and sexual relationships
- Prognosis
- Side-effects of their treatment
- Cancer risk
- Surgery
- Care of young people in transition between paediatric and adult services
- Contact details of support groups.

Crohn's disease is a cause of secondary osteoporosis:

- Do not routinely monitor for changes in bone mineral density in children and young people.
- Consider monitoring for changes in bone mineral density in children and young people with risk factors such as low body mass index, low trauma fracture or continued repeated glucocorticosteroid use.

Give information on pregnancy including the potential risks and benefits of medical treatment and possible effects of Crohn's disease on fertility.

NICE CKS Ulcerative colitis (July 2015)

Managing suspected ulcerative colitis:

In adults:

- Arrange emergency admission if the person has clinical features suggestive of severe ulcerative colitis. These include:
  - more than six stools a day plus at least one of the following features:
    - temperature >37.8°C
    - tachycardia >90bpm
    - anaemia (haemoglobin <10.5g/100ml)
    - ESR >30mm/hour
    - blood in the stool.

- Refer all other people to a gastroenterologist for confirmation of the diagnosis and initiation of treatment.
  - o The urgency of referral will depend on clinical judgement and the severity of symptoms.
  - o Do not offer an anti-diarrhoeal drug (such as loperamide) as it can precipitate toxic megacolon.

Assessing severity of ulcerative colitis

Table 31.1 Truelove and Witts' severity index for assessing severity of ulcerative colitis in adults

	Mild	Moderate	Severe
Bowel movements (number per day)	Fewer than 4	4–6	6 or more plus at least one of the features of systemic upset (marked with * below)
Blood in stools	No more than small amounts of blood	Between mild and severe	Visible blood
Pyrexia (temperature greater than 37.8°C)*	No	No	Yes
Pulse rate greater than 90 beats per minute*	No	No	Yes
Anaemia*	No	No	Yes
Erythrocyte sedimentation rate (mm/hour)*	30 or below	30 or below	Above 30

Available at: http://cks.nice.org.uk/ulcerative-colitis#!scenario

NICE guidelines on ulcerative colitis (CG166, June 2013)

- Discuss the disease and associated symptoms, treatment options and monitoring with person with ulcerative colitis (UC) and their family members or carers as appropriate and within the multidisciplinary team.
- When caring for a pregnant woman with UC, ensure effective communication and information sharing across specialities.
- Consider monitoring bone health in children and young people with UC in the following circumstances: during chronic active disease, after treatment with systemic corticosteroids and after recurrent active disease.
- Monitor height and body weight of children and young people with UC against expected values on centile charts according to disease activity.
- Monitor pubertal development in young people with UC. Consider referral to secondary care paediatrician if patient has slow pubertal progress or has not developed features appropriate for their age.

GP curriculum lists IBD as an important condition that GPs should be familiar with and requires GPs to have an understanding of secondary care management of both Crohn's disease and UC.

Incidence of ulcerative colitis is 6000 to 12,000 per year in the UK and 3000 to 6000 in the UK for Crohn's. Peak age of incidence is 10–40 years. 85% are under the age of 60 years at time of presentation, 10% present under the age of 18 years.

Both UC and Crohn's are chronic, relapsing remitting diseases characterised by acute non-infectious inflammation of the gut. In UC, inflammation is limited to colorectal mucosa; in Crohn's disease, any part of the gut from the mouth to anus can be affected, with normal bowel between affected areas.

Extra-intestinal manifestations (joint, eye and skin disease) are common and both UC and Crohn's disease are risk factors for GI malignancy.

Treatment

Mainstay of treatment of UC is 5-ASA derivative mesalazine. Topical 5-ASA derivatives (rectal mesalazine 1g daily) are a useful adjunct. Steroids (prednisolone) are added if a prompt response is needed.

Infliximab or cyclosporin may be effective as an acute therapy for severe disease; this is specialist-initiated.

Azathioprine is a third-line agent, with surgery being the last resort.

The 5-ASA derivatives such as mesalazine are less effective in Crohn's disease than in UC. Mesalazine is ineffective for maintenance treatment at doses under 2g daily. Flare-ups should be treated with 4g daily. Treatment is aimed at minimising the impact of disease. The most effective measure that patients can take to alleviate the symptoms of Crohn's disease is to stop smoking. Treat diarrhoea symptomatically with codeine phosphate or loperamide unless it is due to active colonic disease.

Steroids are added if active disease is unresponsive to mesalazine.

Help for patients

Information is available from NACC **Crohn's and Colitis UK** (www.crohnsandcolitis. org.uk/). Patients who join are issued with a combined membership and "Can't wait" card. The card carries the message "Please help – our member has a medical condition which means that they need to use your toilet facilities urgently. Your kindness and co-operation would be much appreciated".

The **National Key Scheme** (NKS), previously known as the Royal Association for Disability Rights (RADAR) Scheme, was developed because some public toilets designed for disabled people had to be locked to prevent damage and misuse. This has been countered by their being locked separately from other toilets.

The scheme aims to provide disabled key holders with independent access to the toilets provided for them and increases the likelihood of the facilities being in a usable state.

In addition to public conveniences, toilets for disabled people are provided by a wide range of other public, voluntary and commercial organisations who have joined the scheme, and facilities can now be found in shopping centres, country parks, railway and bus stations, bars, motorway service areas and sports venues. Some local councils will provide this key free, or for a small charge (www.colostomyassociation.org.uk/index.php?p=216...RADAR%20).

Relevant literature

Simon, S (2008) **Inflammatory bowel disease**. *InnovAit*, **1(9)**: 615–622.

CASE 32 Palpitations

INFORMATION FOR THE DOCTOR

Name	Eric Wilton
Age	63
Social and family history	• Married, lives with wife, 2 children aged 14 and 16 • Smokes 20 cigarettes a day • Alcohol 30 units/week • Occupation: taxi driver
Past medical history	• Hay fever, eczema • Oesophagitis with hiatus hernia • SVT, hypertension
Current medication	• Optichrom eye drops PRN • Lansoprazole 30mg OD • Domperidone 10mg TDS • Loratidine 10mg OD • Sotalol 80mg BD • Bendroflumethiazide 2.5mg OD

Letters to GP

Gastroscopy report (4 years ago): Normal gastric mucosa, hiatus hernia and oesophagitis. Advised lansoprazole. No follow-up needed.

ECHO report (2 years ago): Normal LV and RV systolic function. No LV diastolic dysfunction. No LVH. Normal atria size.

INFORMATION FOR THE PATIENT

You are Eric Wilton, a 63-year-old male. You live with your wife and two boys aged 14 and 16 years. You are a taxi driver and work odd shifts. Your wife is a receptionist at a health club.

You are here for routine BP check and repeat prescriptions.

Information to reveal if asked

General information about yourself:

You work odd shifts with a cab company; night shifts pay more. You have several health problems and are on medications for them. You have high blood pressure and it is difficult to make lifestyle changes but you are looking into salt intake and healthier diet.

You also have a history of palpitations, supraventricular tachycardia (SVT) and have been on medications for it. You have been taught certain techniques to control any episodes of palpitations and have had some episodes in the past when you needed to do them. You have had palpitations for two years but started on sotalol six months ago.

You are a smoker, not ready to give up yet. You understand the health risks of smoking and intend to give up in the future.

You binge drink on weekends with friends when you watch football matches at a local pub.

Further details about your condition:

- You ran out of your medications over the weekend when you were visiting your sister for a family function. You indulged in binge drinking and went overboard. You missed all the tablets. You had an episode of palpitations lasting for 2 minutes or so. Your niece is a nurse, who measured your pulse which was 180 beats per minute. You massaged your eyeballs (as you have been instructed to do) and breathed through your closed mouth and nose and the attack subsided. The episode was not associated with chest pains or shortness of breath. You have not had any alcohol since.

- You have had some problems with your circulation lately. You think it started around the time you began the new drug for palpitations.

- You have been having bluish discoloration of finger tips of both hands over 5 months. This was associated with numbness but usually the colour would return to normal quickly.

Your ideas:

- You think you got an attack of your SVT as you missed your medications. You also think that drinking too much without medication could have been a trigger.
- You know there is a problem with your circulation. Your neighbour had suggested discussing the possibility of referral for a scan of the legs. His father had some scans for poor circulation in his legs.

Your concerns:

- You don't have any particular concerns, just want your medications and want to make sure you don't go without them again.

Your expectations:

- You want a repeat prescription for all medications.

Information to reveal if examined

BP: 132/78

P78 regular, heart sounds normal, no murmurs

SUGGESTED APPROACH TO THE CONSULTATION

Targeted history taking:

- Take a detailed history about Eric's palpitations, medication history and details about the recent episode. This should include any red flags like chest pains, syncope, shortness of breath, etc.

- Find out about his vascular problems: this to include any claudication history, colour changes, skin ulcerations, etc.

- Take a social history to include smoking, alcohol and recreational drugs.

Clinical management:

This is a case for medication review.

- The cold hands and feet, with the characteristic colour changes, suggest a diagnosis of Raynaud's disease. Explain Raynaud's to the patient.

- Offer to stop sotalol and evaluate if symptoms improve over the next few weeks.

- As regards treatment of his SVT, ask the patient if he would like to discuss alternative medication now, or if he would like to take some patient information leaflets (on metoprolol and carotid massage) home with him and return to a follow-up appointment later in the week.

- Provide health education regarding smoking and alcohol.

- Give advice about driving and work (see below).

- Address patient's concerns about 'circulation problems' and arrange a referral to rheumatology.

Interpersonal skills:

Good communication with the patient:

- explains his diagnosis of Raynaud's disease in a way the patient understands, discussing treatment and offering drug options.

- checks understanding and offers a follow-up/management plan.

BACKGROUND KNOWLEDGE REQUIRED FOR THIS CASE

One of the side-effects of sotalol (and atenolol) is exacerbation of Raynaud's phenomenon, so a cardio-selective beta-blocker such as metoprolol may be trialled before an alternative treatment for SVT, such as flecainide, which may need initiation under Consultant advice.

Beta-blockers are associated with fatigue and coldness of extremities. They may precipitate asthma and should be avoided in patients with history of asthma or bronchospasm.

The Driver and Vehicle Licensing Agency (DVLA) regulations with regard to palpitations state that:

- For Group 1 entitlement, driving must cease if the arrhythmia has caused or is likely to cause incapacity. Driving may be permitted when the underlying cause has been identified and controlled for at least 4 weeks.

- For Group 2 entitlement, the driver is disqualified from driving if the arrhythmia has caused or is likely to cause incapacity. Driving may be permitted when the arrhythmia is controlled for at least 3 months.

- See the DVLA *At a glance guide to the current medical standards of fitness to drive* (available at www.gov.uk) for further information.

- Those with some occupations, for example people working at height or with potentially dangerous machinery, will need to stop work until a diagnosis is confirmed or the underlying condition is treated.

Table 32.1 Common cardiac arrhythmias

Rhythm	Characteristics	Treatment
Ventricular ectopic beats	These are additional broad QRS complexes without P waves superimposed on a regular sinus rhythm.	Avoidance of caffeine, alcohol, smoking and fatigue. Beta-blockers such as atenolol can be helpful.
Paroxysmal SVT (supraventricular tachycardia)	Common condition, may affect any age group including children. ECG during an attack shows a narrow QRS complex with a regular rate of 130–250bpm.	Carotid sinus massage. Valsalva manoeuvre. Ice on the face. Drugs: IV adenosine or IV verapamil. Recurrent episodes can be treated with catheter ablation or prevented by drugs such as diltiazem, verapamil, flecainide, sotalol or propafenone.
Atrial fibrillation	Characterised by rapid irregularly irregular narrow QRS complex tachycardia with absence of P waves. AF affects in excess of 8% adults aged >60 and is associated with 5× increase in risk of stroke.	Haemodynamically unstable – electrical cardioversion. IV amiodarone or flecainide in non-life-threatening cases when electrical cardioversion delayed. Drugs: beta-blockers, diltiazem (unlicensed indication) or verapamil. Digoxin (used as monotherapy in predominantly sedentary patients). Pharmacological cardioversion amiodarone or flecainide. All patients should be assessed for risk of stroke and need for thromboprophylaxis.

(Continued)

Table 32.1 (Continued)

Rhythm	Characteristics	Treatment
Atrial flutter	ECG shows a regular sawtooth baseline at a rate of 300bpm with narrow QRS complex tachycardia superimposed at a rate of 100 or 150bpm.	Drugs: beta-blockers, diltiazem (unlicensed indication) or verapamil. Digoxin can be added, particularly useful in heart failure patients. Cardioversion: electrical, pharmacological cardioversion or catheter ablation for new atrial flutter. Direct current: needed for rapid conversion, e.g. with haemodynamic compromise.
VT (ventricular tachycardia)	VT causes broad QRS complexes at a rate of 100bpm. VT may be silent or present with palpitations, chest pain, breathlessness and/or collapse.	VT is always a medical emergency. Patient will need oxygen, while awaiting ambulance. Treatment choice: IV amiodarone or lidocaine. If patient has no pulse, should be treated as a cardiac arrest. Pulseless ventricular tachycardia or ventricular fibrillation should be treated with immediate defibrillation. If haemodynamically stable, can be treated with IV anti-arrhythmic drugs. Amiodarone is the preferred drug. Flecainide, propafenone, lidocaine have been used.
Bradycardia Atrioventricular node block or heart block	First-degree block: ECG shows a fixed PR interval of >200ms (1 large square). Second-degree heart block: *Mobitz type I (Wenckebach)*: progressive lengthening PR interval followed by a dropped beat. *Mobitz type II*: ECG shows a constant PR interval with regular dropped beat. Third-degree block: ECG shows P–P interval to be constant and R–R intervals to be constant but not related to each other.	Pacemakers (patient to stop driving for a month after insertion. Patients should inform the DVLA and their insurance company).

Data from *BNF* 68, Sept 2014–15.

Relevant literature

Simon, C (2008) **Palpitations and arrhythmia**. *InnovAiT*, **1(1)**: 25–33.

CASE 33 Falls

INFORMATION FOR THE DOCTOR

You are a doctor making a house call at the request of Rose Thomas, the patient's wife.

Name	Mark Thomas
Age	82
Social and family history	• Married, retired • Alcohol 14 units/week • Ex-smoker
Medical history	• Essential hypertension • Osteoarthritis • Atrial fibrillation • Depression, insomnia • BCC, excised 5 years ago • Shingles
Current medication	• Bendroflumethiazide 2.5mg OD • Fluoxetine 20mg OD • Temazepam 20mg Nocte • Co-dydramol 1–2 tablets QDS/PRN • Simvastatin 20mg Nocte • Digoxin 62.5mg OD • Warfarin 1mg as directed • Warfarin 3mg as directed

INFORMATION FOR THE PATIENT

You are Mrs Rose Thomas, 80-year-old retired librarian, living with your husband Mr Mark Thomas. He is 82 years old, and is a retired builder.

You live together in a bungalow and are completely independent. You have a carer once a week to help with household chores. Your only son lives in Japan. You have requested a home visit for your husband.

Mark has been confused and agitated for a week. You want him to be checked out.

Information to reveal if asked

General information about yourself and Mr Thomas:

- You have been married for 58 years. Your only son Peter has emigrated to Japan. He has married a Japanese girl and lives in Tokyo where he teaches English.

- Mr Thomas manages his weekly shopping, some chores around the house and his finances. His mobility is good and he uses a walking stick. He is hard of hearing and has hearing aids.

Further details about Mr Thomas's condition:

- Confusion has been going on for a week. He has a history of falls and had a fall 10 days ago. You think it was an accidental fall. This happened at night when he needed to use the toilet, forgot to switch on the lights, tripped on the carpet and his slippers and fell over. He managed to get up but had sustained a bruise over his left shoulder and a bump on his head. The pain settled with painkillers which he takes for osteoarthritis. This episode was not associated with chest pains, shortness of breath or loss of consciousness. He hasn't been himself since and is now getting very agitated as well.

Your ideas:

- Mr Thomas has had urinary infections in the past when he has been confused. These have been successfully treated with a course of antibiotics. Urine infection affects his mobility and you think he has come down with another urine infection.

Your concerns:

- You are worried about the worsening of his agitation. He can be difficult to manage and once went off wandering the streets in the middle of the night. Police had to be called and he needed a 2-day stay at the hospital. This was 2 years ago when he had a nasty urine infection. You don't want it to get any worse.

Your expectations:

- You have a urine specimen ready and would like it to be checked and be given a prescription for antibiotics.

- You would agree to get him to hospital for further investigations if needed.

Information to reveal when examined

BP: sitting 138/88, standing 130/86

P86 irregular

HS normal

Chest clear

Urine dip negative

Blood sugar 4.8

Neurology difficult to assess but pupils unequal. Left pupil dilated, reacting poorly to light.

Mini-mental state 5/10. Confused about date/time/place/person/numbers, etc., which is unusual for him. The candidate is not expected to conduct a full mini-mental exam from memory (without aide memoire); simply asking for date/time/place is sufficient questioning.

SUGGESTED APPROACH TO THE CONSULTATION

Targeted history taking:

- Obtain details about the nature of accident or fall to determine if accidental.
- Take a detailed social history about the couple and environmental assessment of their living conditions which may predispose to falls.
- Detail patient's mobility/eyesight, his medical problems and medication history.
- Get details of previous episodes which could point to possible causes.

Targeted examination:

- Examine for blood pressure and pulse; listen to his heart sounds and examine his respiratory system for signs of infection.
- Check for confusion – see if the patient is oriented for date, time, place. Check mobility. Check pupils.
- Dipstix the urine and check his blood sugar.

Clinical management:

- Address Mrs Thomas's concerns about a possible UTI and explain that his condition needs more investigation.
- Arrange an urgent hospital referral for cerebral imaging.
- Medication review is needed as patient has a history of falls and is on warfarin.
- Assess social situation and consider looking into referral for package of care.

This case turned out to be a subdural haematoma.

Interpersonal skills:

Good communication with the patient:

- gives information in a way patient's wife would understand, checks understanding.
- offers support and help which would suit the couple's needs and be acceptable.
- arranges hospital referral and follow-up plans for future care.

This case tests the candidate's ability to conduct a home visit, to assess the patient's capacity and to take a good history from the patient's wife, his primary carer. The doctor's interpersonal skills are tested. The candidate's data-gathering skills are also tested: the ability to risk-assess the possible cause and consequences of the fall. The red flags of confusion and dilated pupils prompt a decision to admit the patient to hospital to exclude a chronic subdural haematoma.

BACKGROUND KNOWLEDGE REQUIRED FOR THIS CASE

Risk factors for falls

Head: cognitive impairment, balance and co-ordination problems, Parkinson's disease, alcohol abuse.

Neck: stiffness, vertebrobasilar insufficiency, carotid sinus hypersensitivity.

Thorax: breathing problems, ischaemia or arrhythmias.

Abdomen: continence problems, diabetes.

Legs: weakness, numbness.

Medication: psychotropic, antihypertensives, anticonvulsants.

Environment: carpets, uneven surfaces, inadequate or inappropriate walking aids, badly-fitting footwear, poor lighting, etc.

Reference: Lawrence, D (2008) **Falls in the elderly**. *InnovAiT*, 1(12), 802–807.

Investigations that may be appropriate

FBC (anaemia or infection), raised MCV (vitamin B12 or folate deficiency or alcohol misuse)

U&E (renal impairment or hyponatraemia)

LFTs, blood glucose (diabetes)

ESR or CRP (polymyalgia rheumatica)

Urinalysis (infection, diabetes)

ECG (AF, bradycardia and conduction defects)

Optician review

Carotid Dopplers, 24-hour tape, cardiac ECHO if symptoms suggestive of TIA

VDRL (syphilis)

CT head

Chest X-ray

DEXA scan for osteoporosis risk

NICE guidelines (CG161, June 2013)
Assessment and prevention of falls in older people

Multifactorial assessment may include the following:

- Identification of falls history
- Assessment of gait, balance, mobility and muscle weakness
- Assessment of osteoporosis risk
- Assessment of the older person's perceived functional ability and fear relating to falling

- Assessment of visual impairment
- Assessment of cognitive impairment and neurological examination
- Assessment of urinary incontinence
- Assessment of home hazards
- Cardiovascular examination and medication review.

Multifactorial interventions. Specific components include:

- Strength and balance training
- Home hazard assessment and intervention
- Vision assessment and referral
- Medication review with modification/withdrawal.

CASE 34 Diarrhoea

INFORMATION FOR THE DOCTOR

Name	Adnan Ghanem
Age	23
Social and family history	• Owner of kebab shop • Non-smoker, teetotaller

INFORMATION FOR THE PATIENT

You are Adnan Ghanem, a 23-year-old Turkish man. You are single and live with your uncle and his family in a 3-bedroom house. Your uncle is married and is 38 years old. His wife is 30 and their two boys are aged 6 and 4 years.

You have been in the UK for four years, have tried several jobs and are now in partnership with your uncle. You and your uncle own a kebab shop and work long hours there.

You have been having diarrhoea for 3 to 4 days. You were reviewed by another GP at the surgery, advised to send a stool sample, have Dioralyte and plenty of fluids.

Information to reveal if asked

General information about yourself:

- You and your uncle own the kebab joint. You got into this partnership 6 months ago and business is really doing well. You make very good money over the weekend.

- You work long hours, sometimes as much as 12–14 hours on the weekends. You take turns with your uncle to look after the shop. You have employed two cooks who are Turkish and have four waiters to help. The venue offers take-away services and has seating availability for up to 20 customers.

- You are currently single, not interested in a relationship or marriage. You want to make enough money to buy your own house.

Further details about your condition:

- Diarrhoea started after having a kebab at work 4 days ago. Loose stools were associated with abdominal cramps and blood but not vomiting. You were feeling very unwell for the first two days – hot and sweaty – but now feel much better. Blood has ceased and now diarrhoea seems to be wearing off.

- You have tried over-the-counter Imodium and Dioralyte, which was recommended by your colleague.

- You have not worked at the kebab shop since the onset of symptoms.

- Another employee, one of the waiters, had similar symptoms and is now off work. He too had food from the shop. He is registered at another practice.

- None of the customers have reported any problems with kebabs or other food. Your uncle and his family are well. They did not consume any of the shop's food.

- The cook had reported a problem with one of the refrigerators which wasn't cooling well. The engineers have been called and the fault is being looked into. Most meat was discarded but some kebabs were thought to be fresh, having just been stored in the fridge the previous morning. These were consumed by you and the waiter who is off sick.

Your ideas:

- You think this is food poisoning.

Your concerns:

- You are worried that you may spread the bug to your uncle's young children. You are being very careful with hand washing and have avoided them completely since the episode.

Your expectations:

- You are here for the stool results and further treatment.

Information to reveal if examined

Abdomen soft, non-tender, no guarding/rigidity

Bowel sounds heard

Temperature 36.2°C

Stool culture:

Cryptosporidium	Not isolated
Campylobacter	Not isolated
E. coli 0157	Positive
Shigella	Not isolated
Salmonella	Not isolated

SUGGESTED APPROACH TO THE CONSULTATION

Targeted history taking:

- Obtains details about the condition, predisposing factors, type of food associated with the diarrhoea.

- Has he travelled abroad recently?

- Has he recently been in contact with anyone else with similar symptoms?

Clinical management:

- Discuss stool results and provide information about *E. coli* gastroenteritis in a way the patient understands.

- Offer symptomatic treatment at this stage and put a follow-up plan in place. Another stool sample to be sent after symptoms have ceased. Stress the importance of avoiding food handling until symptom-free and stool check clear. Other measures to include hand washing, avoiding contact with vulnerable groups.

- Stress the importance of follow-up and/or assessment of his affected employee. His employee needs to see his GP and get a stool culture.

- Advise that any new outbreaks of diarrhoea in connection with the kebab shop to be followed up by suitable health professional.

- Notify health agency, as *E. coli* is a notifiable disease.

Interpersonal skills:

Good communication with the patient:

- gives information in a way patient can understand and checks understanding.

- reassures patient about the nature of problem, yet at same time gives information about possible complications of the infection.

BACKGROUND KNOWLEDGE REQUIRED FOR THIS CASE

Health Protection Agency advice (www.hpa.org.uk)

Certain strains of *E. coli* produce a potent toxin, which causes illnesses ranging from mild diarrhoea through to very severe inflammation of the gut. Occasionally this can cause complications such as kidney failure and anaemia.

Treatment

There is no specific treatment for *E. coli* 0157 infection. Plenty of fluids and rehydration is recommended.

Time away from work or school

Most adults and children over the age of 5 can go back to work or school 48 hours after the first normal stool. Children under 5 should stay away from nurseries and playgroups until they are shown to be completely clear of the bacteria and free from diarrhoea.

Employers must be informed of *E. coli* 0157 infection if handling food, or working with vulnerable groups such as the elderly, the young or people in poor health. In such cases, the affected should stay off work until two further stool tests, at least 48 hours apart, show that the bacteria have cleared.

E. coli 0157 or infectious bloody diarrhoea is a notifiable disease.

List of notifiable diseases (Health Protection Agency 2010)

(www.gov.uk/notifiable-diseases-and-causative-organisms-how-to-report)

Acute encephalitis

Acute infectious hepatitis

Acute meningitis

Acute poliomyelitis

Anthrax

Botulism

Brucellosis

Cholera

Diphtheria

Enteric fever (typhoid or
      paratyphoid fever)

Food poisoning

Haemolytic uraemic syndrome
      (HUS)

Infectious bloody diarrhoea

Invasive group A streptococcal
      disease and scarlet fever

Legionnaires' disease

Leprosy

Malaria

Measles

Meningococcal septicaemia

Mumps

Plague

Rabies

Severe acute respiratory
      syndrome (SARS)

Smallpox

Tetanus

Tuberculosis

Viral haemorrhagic fever (VHF)

Whooping cough

Yellow fever

Reference

www.food.gov.uk/business-industry/guidancenotes/hygguid/foodhandlersguide

CASE 35 Palliative care (low mood)

INFORMATION FOR THE DOCTOR

Name	Frank Page
Age	78
Social and family history	• Married, lives with wife • Has two sons who live abroad • Retired
Past medical history	• Multiple myeloma • Back pain with vertebroplasty 2 years ago • Osteoarthritis • Depression • Gout
Current medication	• Morphgesic SR tablets 30mg BD • Morphgesic SR tablet 10mg BD • Fortisip liquid 200ml TDS • Allopurinol 300mg OD • Lansoprazole 30mg OD • Fluoxetine 20mg OD • Senna 7.5mg OD • Oramorph oral solution 10mg/5ml PRN
Blood tests FBC	*Blood tests done by Macmillan nurse yesterday*
	Hb 9.8g/dL (13.5–18)
	Total WBC 1.8×10^9/L (4–11)
	Monocyte 0.2×10^9/L (0.2–0.8)
	Neutrophil 0.2×10^9/L (2–7.5)
	Basophil 0×10^9/L (<0.1)
	Eosinophil 0.2×10^9/L (0.04–0.4)
	Lymphocytes 1.2×10^9/L (1–4.5)
	Platelet 56×10^9/L (150–400)
U&E	Normal

Recent letters

Consultant haematologist:

> *"I reviewed Mr Page along with his wife in this morning's clinic. He recently had a week on Isle of Wight which was a good break.*

He is now due his 8th cycle (of 10 planned cycles) of treatment with Revlimid for 21 days with dexamethasone for 4 days. His paraprotein is slowly rising and it would appear that Revlimid is holding the disease in check. He has an appointment to see us again in clinic in two months' time."

Mental Health Review:

"Mr Page is known to our services for last two years and has ongoing depression. The main triggers have been his health problems and recent diagnosis of cancer. This has had a major impact on patient and his plans for retired life.

He has received CBT and counselling for it. He continues on 20mg fluoxetine and we will review him in 3 months."

Last consultation with Duty Doctor yesterday:

"Called by Macmillan nurse who is concerned by patient's low mood and tiredness. She has taken a FBC and advised patient to see GP. Appointment booked for tomorrow for face-to-face GP review. Check FBC results."

INFORMATION FOR THE PATIENT

You are Frank Page, a 78-year-old man with multiple myeloma.

You have several health problems and ongoing depression for which you are under the mental health services. You are undergoing chemotherapy for multiple myeloma. You also have ongoing back pain, joint pains and are on potent painkillers for the same. Your mood has gone down since the diagnosis of cancer and you are seeing your doctor for the same.

Your opening statement is *"Good morning, Doctor. I am feeling very low".*

Information to reveal if asked

General information about yourself:

- You live with your wife Rose, aged 76 years, in a 3-bedroom house. You have two sons, one living in New Zealand and the other in the USA. Both are married and settled abroad with their families.

- You are a retired carpenter and were very independent and active before you started the chemotherapy. You enjoyed your DIY, gardening, walking and cycling. Now most of your activities have come to a standstill due to ill health.

Further details about your condition:

- You have finished your 8th cycle of Revlimid. You feel tired, lethargic and hopeless. You had flu last week from which you have been recovering and your morale has hit rock bottom.

- Your back pain was bad enough and now you have to battle with cancer. You think you are the unluckiest guy around.

- Your mood is low, your appetite is poor, you have no interest in any DIY or gardening any more. You feel hopeless and don't care if you don't wake up tomorrow morning. However, you have no thoughts of ending it all.

- Your wife Rose is very supportive, so are your sons. They plan to fly over from New Zealand and the States for Christmas. The worst thing about your diagnosis is that you have had to cancel your cruise which would have marked your 50th wedding anniversary.

- You have had a sore throat which is better, but you still have some generalised body ache.

Your ideas:

- You know it's depression and are on the correct medications for it.

Your concerns:

- You have no fears for yourself, you don't care any more. Sometimes you do worry about Rose and how she will cope after you are gone.

Your expectations:

- You want to know if you could increase the dose of your antidepressants and if it will help.

Information to reveal if examined

Temperature 38°C

Pulse 112bpm

Respiratory rate 22

Chest clear, heart sounds normal

ENT NAD (no abnormality)

SUGGESTED APPROACH TO THE CONSULTATION

Targeted history taking:

- Take detailed history of general condition: tiredness, sore throat, aches and pains.
- Ask him about his depression; mood, appetite, sleep, anhedonia and suicidal ideation.
- Get details of his drug history, including the number of days since his last cycle of chemotherapy.
- Review the FBC results.

Targeted examination:

- General examination to include temperature, pulse, BP, oxygen saturations.
- Cardiovascular, respiratory system and ENT as appropriate.

Clinical management:

- Highlight the importance of your examination findings in relation to patient's recent chemotherapy cycle; assert the need and importance of hospital admission.
- **Arrange urgent hospital admission for neutropenic sepsis.**
- Address patient's mood and related symptoms and discuss his medications/SSRI. Consider an increase in the dose of his antidepressant.
- Arrange a follow-up appointment to assess mood and related symptoms.

Interpersonal skills:

Good communication with the patient:

- shows empathy and hope while discussing his problems.
- checks patient's understanding and offers follow-up appointments.
- discusses any concerns for his elderly wife and offers information and support.

This case tests the doctor's ability to negotiate agendas. The patient has interpreted his increasing tiredness, lethargy and low mood as worsening of his depression. His agenda is to get better treatment for his self-diagnosed worsening depression. The doctor has sight of the patient's recent blood results and is alerted to the possibility of an alternative explanation for his presenting symptoms. If the doctor does not explain his reasons for exploring these alternative explanations, the patient may be left feeling patronised or unheard. A doctor with good interpersonal skills is able to negotiate the agendas and provide information so the patient can re-evaluate his symptoms and hopefully alter his ideas (about the cause of his tiredness and lethargy) and hence his expectations of treatment.

BACKGROUND KNOWLEDGE REQUIRED FOR THIS CASE

NICE (CG151, Sept 2012) *Prevention and management of neutropenic sepsis in cancer patients* (www.nice.org.uk/guidance/cg151)

Provide patients having anticancer treatment and their carers with written and oral information, both before starting and throughout their anti-cancer treatment, on neutropenic sepsis:

- How and when to contact 24 hour specialist oncology advice
- How and when to seek emergency care.

Neutropenic sepsis is a potentially fatal complication of anti-cancer treatment (particularly chemotherapy). Reported mortality rates 2–21%.

Confirming a diagnosis of neutropenic sepsis

Diagnose neutropenic sepsis in patients having anti-cancer treatment whose neutrophil count is 0.5×10^9 per litre or lower and who have:

- a temperature higher than 38°C **or**
- other signs or symptoms consistent with clinically significant sepsis.

Management (Christie Hospital NHS Foundation Trust (2013) Guideline for management of neutropenic sepsis)

Between 50 and 60% of febrile patients prove to have infections and 16–20% of those with a neutrophil count <100/mm³ have bacteraemia. Fever may or may not be present in some infected neutropenic patients who are dehydrated, taking steroids or NSAIDs, and possibility of infection must be considered in any neutropenic patient who is unwell.

Definition of neutropenia

Increased susceptibility to infection is likely when the neutrophil count falls below 1000/mm³ with escalating risk at 500/mm³ and at <100/mm³.

Who to treat

All febrile patients with neutrophil counts <500/mm³ and those whose counts are <1000/mm³ but falling rapidly. Afebrile patients with neutrophil counts <500/mm³ should be treated if they have symptoms compatible with infection.

Sepsis is a systemic inflammatory response syndrome (SIRS) triggered by infection.

SIRS is defined as two or more of the following:

- Temp >38°C or <36°C
- Heart rate >90bpm
- Respiratory rate >20 breaths or $PaCO_2$ <4.3KPa
- WBC $>12 \times 10^9$/L (in those with normal bone marrow activity).

Relevant literature

Cosh, A & Carslaw, H (2013) **What does a GP need to know about chemotherapy?** *InnovAiT*, **6(4)**: 197–205.

CASE 36 Pregnancy care

INFORMATION FOR THE DOCTOR

Name	Nicola Whitehead
Age	40
Social and family history	Teacher, non-smoker, teetotaller, lives with husband
Medical history	• PCOS • Migraines • Hayfever
Current medication	• Rhinolast nasal spray PRN • Sumatriptan 50mg PRN

INFORMATION FOR THE PATIENT

You are Nicola Whitehead, a 40-year-old married woman. You live with your husband. You are a teacher working full-time. You are 31 weeks pregnant.

You suffer from migraines and are here only to collect your repeat prescription.

Your opening statement is *"Can I have a repeat prescription for my sumatriptan please?"*.

Information to reveal if asked

General information about yourself:

- You are 31 weeks pregnant. You love your job as a teacher. You are currently working 40 hours a week. You plan to go on maternity leave at 35 weeks as you have been feeling increasingly tired.

- You plan to have your baby in Spain. Your mother lives in Madrid and you will fly to Spain in the first week of your maternity leave. Your husband plans to join you 3 weeks later if all goes smoothly.

Further details about your condition:

- This is your first pregnancy. You are expecting twins. This is a precious pregnancy as you have conceived after extensive fertility treatments in Spain.

- You had two IVF attempts on the NHS and could not afford private treatment in the UK. Your mother paid for the IVF attempts in Spain. This pregnancy was after your third IVF attempt at a private fertility clinic.

- You will be looked after by the same gynaecology team in the Spanish clinic on your return to Madrid.

- Your fetal scans have been normal. Your midwife check was 3 weeks ago. This was satisfactory.

- You have had a recurrence of headache since last week. This is the first migraine attack since becoming pregnant; the previous one was nearly 10 months ago. The headache itself is not too bad, there are no visual symptoms. No nausea or vomiting. It started as a dull ache seven days ago, is all over your head. The light does not hurt your eyes and you do not have a rash.

- This is not like your usual migraine attack. Your migraines are right-sided headaches and are associated with flashing lights. This is a constant dull headache. It is not very severe like your migraines.

- You usually use paracetamol and Nurofen but occasionally have needed sumatriptan in the past. You tried paracetamol which hasn't helped. You were advised by your Spanish doctor to avoid Nurofen.

Your ideas:

- You think it is your migraine which has presented in an unusual manner. You think this could be related to your pregnancy or hormones.

Your concerns:

- You have a school trip coming up in two days and need to sort out your headache.

Your expectations:

- You want a repeat prescription for sumatriptan.

Medical history

- You have had migraines for years.

- You also had PCOS with irregular periods and fertility problems. There is no history of any ectopic or miscarriages.

Information to reveal if examined

BMI: 38

BP: 183/110. Pedal odema

Urine: Protein +++

Examination: Neurology normal (no abnormalities on fundoscopy); no abdominal tenderness; fetal hearts heard

SUGGESTED APPROACH TO THE CONSULTATION

Targeted history taking:

- Take a history of this pregnancy, the fertility treatment and any past significant gynaecological history.

- Obtain detailed history of headache including previous pattern of headache. Severe or persistent headache? Are there visual abnormalities? Is the headache associated with nausea or vomiting?

- Are there other symptoms such as upper abdominal pain, reduced urination, shortness of breath?

- What are the fetal movements like?

- Is there a family history of pregnancy complications?

Clinical management:

- Discuss the examination finding and its relevance to her pregnancy.

- Address her concerns regarding her migraine and discuss the proposed diagnosis and management of pre-eclampsia.

- Arrange referral to the obstetric unit as per local protocols.

Interpersonal skills:

Good communication with the patient:

- gives information about the proposed diagnosis in simple language, avoiding jargon.

- checks patient understanding.

- agrees on a plan for further management.

Patient was referred to obstetric unit for management of pre-eclampsia.

BACKGROUND KNOWLEDGE REQUIRED FOR THIS CASE

Pre-eclampsia

Pre-eclampsia is pregnancy-induced hypertension in association with proteinuria (more than 0.3g in 24 hours) +/− oedema, and virtually any organ may be affected.

There is consensus that severe hypertension is confirmed with diastolic blood pressure ≥110mmHg on two occasions or systolic blood pressure ≥170mmHg on two occasions and that, together with significant proteinuria (at least 1g/L), this constitutes severe pre-eclampsia.

Risk factors

1. First pregnancy or first pregnancy with a new partner
2. Age 40 or over

3. Pre-eclampsia in previous pregnancies
4. BMI of 35 or more
5. Female relatives (mother/sisters) having a history of pre-eclampsia
6. Multiple births
7. If pregnancy is from egg (oocyte) donation
8. If co-existing medical problems such as high BP, kidney problems and/or diabetes.

Symptoms

Headaches

Blurred vision

Abdominal pain

Nausea/vomiting

Shortness of breath

Confusion

Management

Antihypertensives: treatment should be started in women with systolic BP over 160mmHg or a diastolic BP over 110mmHg.

Methyldopa and labetalol are the most commonly used therapies in the UK. Labetalol is given orally or IV. Nifedipine given orally or hydralazine IV for acute management.

Atenolol, ACE inhibitors, ARB and diuretics should be avoided.

Nifedipine should not be given sublingually, but orally instead.

Arrange urgent obstetric admission if any of the following criteria are met:

- Urine dipstick testing is positive for 1+ or more protein.
- She has symptoms of pre-eclampsia.
- Blood pressure is 160/110mmHg or higher.

NICE recommends that all women with gestational hypertension/pre-eclampsia should be offered an integrated package of care that may include hospital admission, regular measurement of blood pressure, testing for proteinuria, and relevant blood tests. Admission to hospital is recommended if blood pressure is 160/110mmHg or greater.

Relevant literature

RCOG Guideline No10 (A)

www.rcog.org.uk/en/patients/patient-leaflets/pre-eclampsia/

NICE (2011) *Hypertension in pregnancy – the management of hypertensive disorders during pregnancy.*

CASE 37 Sick note (transsexuality)

INFORMATION FOR THE DOCTOR

Name	Jerry Parker
Age	52
Social and family history	• Works in a superstore • Non-smoker, social drinker • Lives with partner
Past medical history	• Type 1 diabetes • Hypercholesterolaemia • Hypertension • CKD3 • TIA (3 years ago) • Gender reassignment surgery (combined operation transformation male to female) • Eczema
Current medication	• Ramipril 5mg OD • Novorapid penfill inj. sol. 100 units/ml • Lantus cartridge inj. sol. 100 units/ml • Premarin tablet 1.25mg OD • Aspirin 75mg OD • Hydrocortisone 1% cream PRN • Diprobase 500ml cream BD
Blood results FBC U&E LFTs Lipid profile	Hb 13.8g/dL HbA1c 48 WBC 4.4×10^9/L Platelet 222×10^9/L Na 140mmol (135–145) K 4.0 (3.2–5.0) Cr 77µmol/L (44–80) Urine albumin 7.3mg/L Urine creatinine 11.0 ACR 0.7mg/mmol Alk. phos. 72IU/L (35–104) T. bilirubin 13µmol/L (0.0–21.0) Al. aminotransferase 19.0 (0.0–31.0) Total cholesterol 6.8mmol/L (2.8–5) LDL 3.2mmol/L (0.0–3.0) Triglyceride 2.1mmol/L (0.8–1.7)

Recent A&E letter

> *"Patient attended the department after an accidental fall, sustained a right ankle injury. X-ray ruled out fractures. She has been discharged, recommended rest/ice packs/leg elevation."*

INFORMATION FOR THE PATIENT

You are Jerry Parker, a 52-year-old female (you had a gender reassignment surgery to change from male to female).

You live with your male partner Dylan Jackson and your two cats in a rented flat.

You work in a superstore. Your partner drives a cab.

You had a fall a few days ago and are here for a sick note.

Your opening statement is *"Doctor, I need a sick note and repeat prescriptions please".*

Information to reveal if asked

General information about yourself:

- You work in a superstore and have a physical job. You stack shelves and are responsible for checking supplies, assisting in storage, etc. You work full-time for 40 hours a week.

- You are in a stable relationship. You met your current partner in the bar where he worked 2 years ago. He now works as a taxi driver. He knows about your gender reassignment and there are no issues about it.

- Your gender reassignment surgery happened 7 years ago and you think it was the most liberating experience. The procedure itself was a two-step operation but you went through it and have never been happier. You always thought you were a woman trapped in a man's body and this was the only way out. Your family – your mother and sister – had reservations at first but now they are very happy for you.

Further details about your condition:

- You sustained a right ankle injury when you tripped on a pavement. This happened six days ago when it was raining and the roads were slippery. You were wearing high heels and were walking on a steep pavement.

- Your job involves stacking shelves and moving goods. You would like to have a sick note as your manager can be 'fussy'. Otherwise things are fine. The injury has incapacitated you but Dylan is very supportive. He has flexible working hours and does all the chores.

- Your right ankle is swollen and painful but you are taking paracetamol and ibuprofen which seem to control the pain.

- You had a mini stroke (TIA) three years ago. The episode was marked with slurred speech and confusion lasted for 30 minutes. You were investigated, were commenced on aspirin and have been fine since.

- You are not keen on statins as they have given you muscle cramps in the past, and you will try to control cholesterol with lifestyle management. Your diabetes is well under control with no related problems.

- There have been issues about the Premarin in the past. The consultant at the TIA clinic and your previous GPs have discussed the risks associated with use of Premarin. You would rather risk a stroke than lose your femininity. You have gone to great lengths to be a woman and are not willing to stop Premarin.

Your ideas:

- You know about the management of your ankle injury and are doing everything that A&E recommended. You are also aware about the risks involved with use of Premarin and further risk of stroke but are willing to take the risk.

Your concerns:

- You have no particular concerns.

Your expectations:

- You want a sick note for 2 weeks.

- You also want a repeat prescription for your insulins, aspirin and Premarin.

Information to reveal if examined

BMI 22

BP normal

Right ankle swollen, no bony tenderness on calcaneus or malleoli.

SUGGESTED APPROACH TO THE CONSULTATION

Targeted history taking:

- Obtains details about her medical problems and medications. This is to include details about her gender reassignment, TIA history and diabetes.
- Takes a detailed history of the fall and any history of possible hypoglycaemic episodes which could have contributed to the accident.
- What is her social history, lifestyle, diet, alcohol and smoking history?

Targeted examination:

- Ankle examination
- BP, BMI

Clinical management:

- Discuss the risks and complications of use of HRT with history of stroke. This patient is on Premarin. Discuss the possibility of changing to oestradiol patch 25–50µg twice weekly, which may improve her CV risk profile while maintaining a feminising effect.
- Discuss lifestyle changes to reduce cholesterol level. This should include diet and exercise.
- Discuss other options including possibility of statin or other cholesterol-reducing drugs.
- Fulfil expectation of a sick note and issue of repeat prescriptions.

Interpersonal skills:

Good communication with the patient:

- works with the patient, respects her choice and decisions to continue with HRT.
- is non-judgemental about her lifestyle and offers information and options in a way the patient will understand.

BACKGROUND KNOWLEDGE REQUIRED FOR THIS CASE

This case has complex issues about gender identity and risks involved with oestrogen use. It is about patient education and choice.

Non-oral oestrogens, including sublingual, transdermal, and injectable hormones, are preferable to oral preparations as these have the advantage of avoiding first pass through liver metabolism.

- Dosing: sublingual (dissolve oral formulation under the tongue) 1–4mg estradiol/day (single or divided dose), 100–200mcg transdermal estradiol/day, 10–20mg estradiol valerate IM every 1–2 weeks (injections continue for no more than 2 years, then change to lower dosage).

- Over 35/smokers: oral oestrogens (estradiol 0.5–2mg OD, BD or TDS) confer an increased risk of thromboembolic disease.
- After gonadectomy: lower doses are recommended: 50–100mcg transdermal, 1–2mg sublingual estradiol. Titrate the dose to effect, considering patient tolerance.

  From http://transhealth.ucsf.edu/trans?page=protocol-hormones

Relevant literature

BNF (Sept 2014–March 2015)

www.gires.org.uk/assets/DOH-Assets/pdf/doh-guidelines-for-clinicians.pdf

CASE 38 Shortness of breath

INFORMATION FOR THE DOCTOR

You are a doctor on a home visit.

Name	Paul Spiers
Age	70
Social and family history	• Retired, non-smoker, social drinker • Lives with wife • Has been living in the UK/Cyprus for last 2 years
Past medical history	• Depression • Type 2 diabetes • Atrial fibrillation • Erectile dysfunction • Gastro-oesophageal reflux • Herpes zoster
Current medication	• Venlafaxine 150mg OD • Omeprazole 20mg OD • Simvastatin 40mg Nocte • Warfarin 5mg as directed • Warfarin 3mg as directed • Ramipril 2.5mg OD • Atenolol 50mg OD

Cardiology report (2 years ago)

Diagnosis: atrial fibrillation, cardioverted to sinus rhythm.

ECHO – mild systolic impairment, ejection fraction 51% with dilated LA. Mild AS, mild AR. Follow-up with consultant in 2 weeks.

Notes from appointment one week ago with practice nurse for chronic disease monitoring

Patient has diet-controlled type 2 diabetes and takes medication for hypertension and AF, but has been seen in Cyprus recently for treatment. Says he is compliant on medication. Attends later for blood tests & BP check prior to seeing GP next week for a repeat prescription of medication. He reports some mild breathlessness but no chest pain on exertion and the duty doctor (Dr Bajaj) advised me to also request BNP as well as routine diabetic bloods.

Blood tests	Blood tests done recently
FBC	normal
HbA1c	6.9g%
Fasting cholesterol	4.2mmol/L
Fasting HDL cholesterol	1.0mmol/L (0.8–1.8)
TSH	2.75 (0.35–5.5)
Alkaline phosphatase	279IU/L (95–280)
Total bilirubin	11µmol/L (3–17)
Albumin	42g/L (35–50)
Creatinine level	104µmol/L (70–150)
U&Es	within the normal range
BMI	27
BNP	432pg/ml
	(high >400pg/ml, raised 100–400pg/ml, normal <100pg/ml)

INFORMATION FOR THE PATIENT

You are Paul Spiers, a 70-year-old retired teacher. You live with your wife. You have a house in Cyprus and have been living there with occasional visits to the UK.

You have few medical problems but have been keeping well and were looked after by a local GP in Cyprus. You did not have any regular follow-ups by the GP in Cyprus, and only attended surgery for minor ailments. You were taking the UK equivalent of your medications in Cyprus but have re-registered with your previous practice.

Information to reveal if asked

General information about yourself:

- You returned to the UK last month and plan to be here for at least 6 months as there is a lot of unfinished business. You have two houses which you now plan to put on the market. You intend to buy a retirement flat, sort out your will and some other financial issues, and return to Cyprus in a few months.
- You have a son who is an accountant and lives in Scotland.

Further details about your condition:

- You have requested a home visit as you have been feeling very breathless and exhausted. You were not able to keep any hospital appointments for last 2 years due to lifestyle and travel. You did get a letter at your UK address from cardiology last year but were not able to attend. Your warfarin was monitored on and off and you have somehow managed.
- Your last hospital appointment was with a heart specialist, when you had some scans and were diagnosed with a fast heart rate. You did not keep the follow-up appointment.
- You have been getting increasingly short of breath on walking a few steps in the house. Your feet have got puffy and you need to sleep in an armchair. You have had no chest pains or palpitations.

Your ideas:

- You know it's a heart problem as you were told there was a leak in one of your valves.

Your concerns:

- You are worried that your heart should not deteriorate or stop before you finish your planned ventures in the UK.

Your expectations:

- You are happy to be referred back to the heart specialist. You promise compliance this time.
- You want to know what is the diagnosis and any complications of your heart problem.

Information to reveal if examined

Cardiovascular examination:

BP 180/101

P88 regular

PO_2 – 94%

Oedema up to the knees

Heart sounds normal with bilateral basal crepitations.

SUGGESTED APPROACH TO THE CONSULTATION

Targeted history taking:

- Obtain details about his main symptoms – what made him request a home visit today? How severe is his breathlessness? Is there any illness (acute coronary syndrome, infection) that could have led to a deterioration in his condition?
- Ask about Mr Spiers' lifestyle, smoking, alcohol and activity levels and ability.
- Take a detailed history of his cardiac and respiratory symptoms.

Clinical management:

- Discuss the diagnosis and management of his condition in a way he understands.
- He is already on an ACE inhibitor (consider increasing the dose and checking renal function in 7–10 days). Consider whether furosemide 40mg twice daily may be useful to help with breathlessness, or if spironolactone or hydralazine may be a better long-term choice.
- He is on atenolol, but bisoprolol 1.25mg once daily may be a better option.
- Arrange a hospital referral and cardiology follow-up as per local protocol. As his BNP is >400pg/ml, he requires an echocardiogram in secondary care (within two weeks as recommended by NICE).
- Arrange follow-up to improve his BP, AF and diabetic control.

Patient was referred to hospital for management of heart failure.

Interpersonal skills:

Good communication with the patient:

- discusses his diagnosis in a way he understands.
- offers referral to specialist units and follow-up in surgery for further management.

This case tests the candidate's ability to make a diagnosis of heart failure and to explain the condition and management plan (cardiology referral) to the patient. The patient's clinical condition has deteriorated since he was seen last week in surgery, so the candidate has to make a decision about whether to initiate any drug treatment to help resolve or reduce symptoms while the patient awaits cardiology assessment.

BACKGROUND KNOWLEDGE REQUIRED FOR THIS CASE

NICE guidelines (highlights) (CG108, August 2010)
Diagnosing heart failure

Measure serum natriuretic peptides (B type natriuretic peptide BNP) or N-terminal pro-B type natriuretic peptide (NTproBNP) in patients with suspected heart failure without previous MI.

If suspected heart failure and previous MI, patients need transthoracic Doppler 2D echocardiography and specialist assessment within 2 weeks.

Very high levels of serum natriuretic peptides carry a poor prognosis. Refer patients with suspected heart failure and a BNP level above 400pg/ml or NTproBNP level above 2000pg/ml (236pmol/L) urgently to have echocardiography and specialist assessment within 2 weeks.

Refer patients with suspected heart failure and a BNP level between 100 and 400pg/ml or an NTproBNP level between 400 and 2000pg/ml to have echocardiography and a specialist assessment within 6 weeks.

Serum natriuretic peptides

Obesity, diuretics, ACE/ARBs, beta-blockers and aldosterone antagonists can reduce levels.

High levels can have other causes such as: age >70, liver cirrhosis, sepsis, COPD, left ventricular hypertrophy.

Treatment

Lifestyle advice for heart failure patients and other issues which need to be discussed:

- Exercise: offer a supervised group exercise-based rehabilitation programme designed for patients with heart failure
- Smoking: strongly advise against smoking
- Alcohol: abstain from drinking alcohol
- Sexual activity: discuss these sensitive issues with patient
- Vaccination: annual vaccination against influenza and pneumococcal disease
- Air travel: depends on their clinical condition at time of travel.

Drugs:

- ACE inhibitors and beta-blockers licensed for heart failure as first-line treatment (bisoprolol, carvedilol). Nebivolol is licensed for stable mild to moderate heart failure. ARB if intolerant to ACE.
- Aldosterone antagonist (spironolactone) licensed for moderate to severe heart failure or MI in past month (can consider in those who are already taking ACE).
- Hydralazine in combination with nitrate (especially in people of African or Caribbean origin with moderate to severe heart failure).

Relevant literature

NICE CG 108 (August 2010) *Chronic heart failure: management of chronic heart failure in adults in primary and secondary care.*

CASE 39 Chronic disease management

INFORMATION FOR THE DOCTOR

Name	Mark Wood
Age	42
Social and family history	• Smoker (15 cigarettes/day) • Alcohol 12 units/week • Manager, sports retail chain • Married, lives with wife and two young sons
Blood tests TSH Free T$_4$ Alanine aminotransferase Total bilirubin Alk phosphatase Globulin Plasma glucose Creatinine Potassium Sodium Total cholesterol Triglyceride HDL cholesterol LDL cholesterol Hb WBC Platelet	*Blood tests done recently* 2.64mIU/L (<5) 12.4pmol/L (12–22) 36.0 (0–42) 4μmol/L (<21) 61IU/L (40–129) 30g/L 5mmol/L 84μmol/L (62–106) 3.9mmol/L (3.2–5.0) 137mmol/L (135–145) 9.6mmol/L (2.8–5.0) 11.1mmol/L (0.8–1.7) 1.0mmol/L (≥1.0) 4.9mmol/L (0–3.0) 14.1g/L 6.3 × 10^9/L 230 × 10^9/L

INFORMATION FOR THE PATIENT

You are Mark Wood, a 42-year-old male. You are married and live with your wife and sons in your four-bedroom house.

You are a manager of a sports shop and work long hours. Your wife works part-time. She is an optician. You have sons aged 7 and 9 years.

You are here for your blood tests. This is the first time you have had a blood test as a routine check. Some colleagues at work were having theirs done and you thought it might be a good idea.

Information to reveal if asked
General information about yourself:
- You are a manager of a sport retail chain and manage four stores in the area. This is a very busy job and can be highly pressured in today's competitive world.
- You work long hours and often work on weekends, so do not have much time for hobbies or exercise. Work can be stressful and whatever free time you have is taken up by your young children.
- Two of your colleagues were having a routine check which involved blood tests and other checks. You decided to have one for yourself as well. You are otherwise well in yourself with no complaints.

Further details about your condition:
- You have a heavy breakfast, usually fried stuff which you love. Your breakfast can vary between double omelette, toast, sausages, hash browns and coffee. Lunch can be fish and chips at a local shop or pasta and related meals if at a meeting. Dinners are home-cooked, usually vegetables and some form of white meat or fish.
- There is strong family history of cardiac problems. Your brother, living in the USA, recently had a heart attack at 45 years of age. He was found to have high cholesterol and has been commenced on medications for it. Your father died of a heart attack at 49 years; he was never investigated. Your mother is well.
- You are realistic that you are unable to make many lifestyle changes and are happy to start medications for your cholesterol. If counselled about risk factors, you will agree to consider smoking cessation.
- You will agree to have genetic tests for any familial conditions of high cholesterol as this could be relevant to your children. If offered a genetic test, you will be happy to consider it.
- You will want to know if your children need testing if you have a 'positive' test to any familial condition.

- You work long hours in an office-based job with not much physical activity during the day.

Your ideas:

- You know you don't have a very healthy lifestyle and won't be surprised to know that you could have high cholesterol.

Your concerns:

- You have been worried about your heart since your brother had his heart attack 18 months ago. You would rather take steps to prevent such an emergency.

Your expectations:

- You are here for the blood results and want to know the next step in keeping well.

Social history

You have tried to give up smoking in the past but failed. Your wife keeps nagging you about giving it up as you have two young sons. You can consider smoking cessation in the future.

You are a social drinker.

Information to reveal if examined

BP 128/78

P76, Chest clear, HS normal

No tendon exanthomata

SUGGESTED APPROACH TO THE CONSULTATION

Targeted history taking:

- Take a detailed history of Mark's lifestyle. This should include dietary history, his levels of activity or exercise, smoking and alcohol status.

- Obtain a detailed family history in relation to cardiac problems, strokes or related conditions.

- Examine for tendon exanthomata.

Clinical management:

- Discuss his blood tests – cholesterol is raised, and raised to the extent to suggest the possibility of familial hypercholesterolaemia, an autosomal dominant genetic condition putting him at risk of early CV disease. A 2nd blood test is needed to confirm cholesterol levels and if they are high, referral to lipid clinic, cardiology, genetic clinic, or a dietician may be needed (as per local protocol).

- Discuss treatment of the high cholesterol, with diet and statins. The patient may want further information on the risks, benefits and monitoring of lipids while on lipid lowering medication, so consider a patient information leaflet.

- In view of his family history of early MI, organise an ECG and consider referral to cardiology.

- Share the BP results with the patient and inform him that as long as his BP remains below 140/90, he does not require anti-hypertensive medication.

- As long as his HbA1c is <42 or fasting glucose <6, he does not require medication for diabetes.

Interpersonal skills:

Good communication with the patient:

- Discusses blood results and gives information in a way patient can understand.

- Offers options of medical and non-medical management, seeks patient's decision.

- Comes up with a shared management plan and offers follow-ups.

BACKGROUND KNOWLEDGE REQUIRED FOR THIS CASE

NICE CG 71 (August 2008) Quick reference guide (Familial hypercholesterolaemia)

Familial hypercholesterolaemia (FH) is a genetic condition that causes high cholesterol concentration in blood. The disease is transmitted in a dominant pattern and siblings and children of a person with FH have a 50% risk of inheriting FH.

Having this condition leads to a greater than 50% risk of coronary heart disease in men by age 50 and at least 30% in women by age 60, if left untreated.

Consider the possibility of FH in adults who have raised total cholesterol concentrations (typically greater than 7.5mmol/L), especially if there is a personal or family history of premature coronary heart disease.

Simon Broome Diagnostic Criteria for Index Individuals

Diagnose a person with definite FH if they have cholesterol concentrations as defined

	Total cholesterol	LDL-C
Child/young person	>6.7mmol/L	>4.0mmol/L
Adult	>7.5mmol/L	>4.9mmol/L

and tendon xanthomas or evidence of these signs in first- or second-degree relative

or

DNA-based evidence of an LDL-receptor mutation, familial defective apo B-100, or a PCSK9 mutation.

Diagnose a person with possible FH if they have cholesterol concentrations as defined in the table above and at least one of the following:

Family history of myocardial infarction: aged <50 in second-degree relative or aged <60 in first-degree relative.

Family history of raised total cholesterol: >7.5mmol/L in adult first- or second-degree relative or >6.7mmol/L in child, brother or sister aged <16.

Offer DNA test to people with clinical diagnosis of FH.

Do not use coronary heart disease risk estimation tools, such as those based on Framingham algorithm, because people with FH are already at high risk of premature coronary heart disease.

When offering lipid-modifying drug therapy, inform that this treatment will be lifelong.

Additional information

www.geneticseducation.nhs.uk/downloads/0066Patients_experiences_report_Sept_2007.pdf (page 41)

www.geneticseducation.nhs.uk/for-practitioners-62/clinical-management/referalls

http://cks.nice.org.uk/hypercholesterolaemia-familial#!scenario

CASE 40 Urinary tract infection

INFORMATION FOR THE DOCTOR

Name	Megan Smith
Age	23
Social and family history	Smokes 10 cigarettes/day, social drinker
Medical history	• Chlamydia a year ago: treated with azithromycin • UTIs – 4 episodes: treated with trimethoprim • Vaginal thrush: treated with Canesten
Current medication	Cerazette

INFORMATION FOR THE PATIENT

You are Megan Smith, a 23-year-old female. You work as a waitress. You share a flat with three flatmates.

You are a smoker (up to 10 cigarettes a day), and are a social drinker, drinking when you go out on weekends.

You are currently single. You don't have a regular partner but have been out with several men in the past few months. Two of them work in the same café as you, while another one is an old friend with whom you have had an on and off relationship.

You are prone to urine infections and need antibiotics for them. You are here at the doctors for a urine infection.

Your opening statement is *"Doctor I think it's bad cystitis again".*

Information to reveal if asked

- After leaving school, you have tried several jobs, and are currently working in a café.

- You live with friends. You don't have a regular partner. You have been in a relationship in the past; he is now a good friend and you see him on and off. He is not your boyfriend any more but you have a sexual relationship with him.

- You have also had flings with two other men who work with you but this was a one off. Your partners have never used condoms.

- You are on the pill but have been a bit forgetful about it. You are unsure if you could have missed any in the last few weeks. You don't get periods on the mini pill.

- You have been experiencing lower abdominal pain, feeling a bit dizzy and you are not sure if there has been blood in your urine. You sometimes spot on your Pill and there has been some spotting 'down below'. You had nausea but no hot or cold spells or temperature symptoms. You have not had a vaginal discharge.

- You have been having lower abdominal pain since last evening. Pains have now got worse, you feel nauseous but you haven't vomited. You don't have any urgency or frequency of urination. The pain is over your lower right abdomen.

Further details about your condition:

- You are prone to urine infections. You have had four infections in the last six months. You have some urgency and frequency of micturition but no blood on this occasion. On one occasion you had severe lower abdominal pains and blood in your urine.

- You have a busy lifestyle. You work as a waitress in a café, where shifts can be long without breaks. Some days you work for twelve hours with only two breaks in between. You have been making a conscious effort to drink fluids frequently and have regular toilet breaks. You are also trying cranberry juice which was recommended by your flatmate.

Your ideas:

- You think it is cystitis as you are prone to it. You have taken 'cystitis' sachets given by the pharmacist but this has not helped.

Your concerns:

- You don't want it to get worse as you have a busy week ahead. This time the pain is severe enough to make you take a day off from work and attend the surgery.

Your expectations:

- You want antibiotics again.

Information to reveal if examined

Urine dip positive leucocytes, negative for nitrites and blood

Suprapubic tenderness and marked tenderness in right iliac fossa

P 112

BP 128/78

Temp 36.2°C

Pregnancy test positive

SUGGESTED APPROACH TO THE CONSULTATION

Targeted history taking:

- Take a detailed history of symptoms: abdominal pain, PV bleeding and nausea. Compare these symptoms with previous 'cystitis' symptoms and note the absence of frequency and dysuria.

- Obtain a menstrual history and sexual history. This should also include details of contraception, any missed pills and use of condoms during sexual encounters.

- Risk assess for ectopic pregnancy and STI. Has she had previous chlamydia infection, tubal surgery, IUD or POP use, fertility treatment or previous ectopic pregnancy?

Clinical management:

- Address patient's concerns about possible urinary tract infection and inform her about the possible diagnosis.

- Discuss the diagnosis and give information in a way she understands. Arrange urgent referral to the hospital for suspected ectopic pregnancy.

- Discuss risks of STI and offer follow-up.

Interpersonal skills:

Good communication with the patient:

- is non-judgemental about patient's lifestyle and sexual history.

- is empathetic and discusses treatment options. Be prepared to answer questions on investigations (transvaginal ultrasound and hCG) and treatment (conservative, surgical or medical).

- checks patient's understanding and offers follow-up to plan for future successful contraception or pregnancies. Having had one ectopic, the risk of having another is 15%. Consider an early scan in a subsequent pregnancy.

BACKGROUND KNOWLEDGE REQUIRED FOR THIS CASE

- Suspect an ectopic pregnancy in any woman with a positive pregnancy test and abdominal pain or GI symptoms, unless ultrasound has already confirmed intrauterine pregnancy.

- Most ectopics will rupture before 8 weeks of gestation, when their size can no longer be contained by the Fallopian tube. Ectopic is rare if gestation is reliably over 10 weeks.

- With pregnancy testing as sensitive as it is now, it is impossible for a woman to have an ectopic pregnancy without the pregnancy test being positive.

- Most suspected ectopic pregnancies can be referred to the next available early pregnancy clinic appointment, unless the patient has severe pain or is cardiovascularly compromised.
- A combination of serum hCG and transvaginal ultrasound is needed for diagnosis. This is offered in the early pregnancy clinic.
- If a patient shows signs of haemodynamic instability, surgical management is the only option.

Risk factors

Previous ectopic

Damaged Fallopian tubes

IUD

POP or mini pill

IVF or ICSI

Age >40 years

Smokers

Symptoms

Abnormal bleeding, pain in lower abdomen or tip of the shoulder, diarrhoea or pain on opening bowels and occasionally severe pain with collapse.

The overall chance of having an ectopic pregnancy next time is 7–10%.

Relevant literature

Royal College of Obstetricians and Gynaecologists patient information leaflet, August 2010 (www.rcog.org.uk/globalassets/documents/patients/patient-information-leaflets/pregnancy/pi-an-ectopic-pregnancy.pdf)

The Ectopic Pregnancy Trust: www.ectopic.org.uk

CASE 41 Genetics

INFORMATION FOR THE DOCTOR

Name	Gisela Sanchez
Age	26
Social and family history	• Professional ballet dancer • Non-smoker, vegetarian • Married, lives with husband and daughter aged 4 years.

Letter from metabolic unit

Diagnosis: CPT-2 deficiency (carnitine palmitoyltransferase type 2 deficiency)

Medications: Coenzyme Q10 100mg TDS

> *Dear Doctor,*
>
> *Thanks for the referral of your 26-year-old patient who is a professional ballet dancer. As you are aware, she has been having intermittent episodes of muscle pain and weakness dating back to childhood. She has had numerous investigations over the years and CPT-2 deficiency was recently confirmed by fibroblast studies, reduced enzyme activity and mutation analysis.*
>
> *CPT-2 deficiency has autosomal recessive inheritance and characteristic symptoms include rhabdomyolysis, myoglobinuria and recurrent myalgia.*
>
> *Gisela has been dancing seriously for last 2 years and her symptoms have worsened. They involve lower limbs and neck. She has had three hospital admissions with acute crises generally due to fever and physical exertion.*

Treatment options include high carbohydrate/low fat diet, trial of benzafibrate 200mg TDS. She can be referred to local genetics team for counselling.

INFORMATION FOR THE PATIENT

You are Gisela Sanchez, a 26-year-old female. You are married and live with your husband and your 4-year-old daughter.

You are a professional ballet dancer. You have stage performances in Europe and America and are very busy managing your career and home.

Your dance has taken a toll on your health and you have been feeling tired and exhausted lately. You had been hospitalised for exhaustion and hence were being investigated for some muscle problems. You saw a specialist at a metabolic unit who had suggested genetic tests which could explain the problems with your muscles and your fatigue.

You are here for the test results, some of which were genetics tests sent to a specialised unit.

Your opening statement is *"Doctor I need to discuss my results".*

Information to reveal if asked

General information about yourself:

- You are a ballet dancer and dance is your passion. You are at the peak of your career and you need to practise daily for long hours. You have been feeling tired and exhausted lately as you have been putting in extra effort for the forthcoming shows.
- Your husband is an IT professional, is able to work from home and is very supportive. He manages the house and childcare when you are busy or touring.

Further details about your condition:

- You are Spanish, the eldest of four daughters. Your youngest sister is being investigated for similar symptoms in Spain. Your parents are first cousins. Your husband is German; you are unrelated.
- You seemed to have leg aches even as a child. Sometimes these aches and pains would last for days and these were related to any physical activity.
- Your mother was a dancer but she never had any problems. Two of your sisters are pursuing dance.
- You know of the genetic disorder and its implications. The specialist briefly discussed the possibility of you having an enzyme deficiency. You have read a lot about it on the internet.
- The specialist has recommended an alternative career but ballet is your 'life'. You practise five to six hours a day and are rehearsing for a performance in 8 weeks in New York. This is something you have looked forward to all your life, but you

may think of cutting down after the show. You have been offered a position of a dance teacher in a private school and will think about it.

Your ideas:

- You know this is a genetic problem and the specialist had discussed it in detail before sending off bloods and other investigations. You have read a lot about it and have realised that all your symptoms fit into this deficiency.

Your concerns:

- You are concerned about your daughter inheriting the disorder. The specialist did not discuss that aspect of the problem and you want to know what her chances are of having the condition if your test results are positive.

Your expectations:

- You are here for your results. You want to know if you have 'CP-2 deficiency' and the chances that your daughter might have it.

SUGGESTED APPROACH TO THE CONSULTATION

Targeted history taking:

- Obtain details about her symptoms, any serious complications in relation to the episodes.

- Take a detailed family history about any other family members having similar problems. This history should include a family tree with affected members and details about marriage between cousins, etc.

Clinical management:

- Inform patient about the diagnosis which has been confirmed by genetic testing.

- Discuss a management plan for any future episodes of fatigue, exhaustion or muscle pains.

- Address patient's concerns about the risk to her child and discuss mode of inheritance in a manner she would understand.

Interpersonal skills:

Good communication with the patient:

- gives information in a way the patient will understand in simple language with frequent checking of patient's understanding.

This case tests the ability of the doctor to read and understand the information presented in a consultant's letter and then use this information to address any questions that the patient has. The temptation in this consultation is to make assumptions about the patient's expectations and to stick to the facts about the medical condition without exploring the psycho-social fallout. This is a presentation about loss – this young patient has received news about an illness and has to process how this will affect her dance which is both her passion, livelihood and source of esteem. She may be worried about passing 'bad' genes to her daughter, so guilt may also be tied up with feelings of loss, disempowerment and fear. A holistic and caring doctor not only attends to her physical needs, but is also present for her emotionally. Active listening, therapeutic validation and empathy are needed.

BACKGROUND KNOWLEDGE REQUIRED FOR THIS CASE

Autosomal dominant inheritance

Males and females affected in equal proportions

Transmitted from one generation to next (vertical transmission)

All forms of transmission are observed (i.e. male to male, female to female and male to female)

Autosomal recessive inheritance

Males and females are affected in equal proportions

Siblings of an affected individual have a 1:4 chance of being affected

Consanguinity in the parents provides further support

X-linked recessive inheritance

Males affected almost exclusively

Transmitted through carrier females to their sons ('knight move' pattern)

Affected males cannot transmit the disorder to their sons.

X-linked dominant inheritance

Males and females are affected but affected females occur more frequently than affected males.

Females are usually less severely affected than males.

While affected females can transmit the disorder to male and female children, affected males transmit the disorder only to their daughters, all of whom are affected.

Other key points

If all children of affected mothers are affected, but no children of affected fathers, consider the possibility of mitochondrial inheritance.

If there are children with multiple malformations and stillbirths in several generations, consider the possibility of the family having a chromosomal translocation.

Relevant literature

Simon, C and Farndon, P (2008) **What causes genetic disorders?** *InnovAiT*, **1(8)**: 544–553.

http://mh.bmj.com/content/30/2/63.full

CASE 42 Carpal tunnel syndrome

INFORMATION FOR THE DOCTOR

Name	Anita Savage
Age	52
Social and family history	• Married, lives with husband and two sons aged 13 and 15 years • Occupation: computer programmer • Non-smoker, social drinker
Blood tests U&E LFTs Fasting BM TSH T$_4$ BMI BP	*Blood tests done recently* normal normal 5.0 10mIU/L (<5mIU/L) 6pmol/L (12.0–22.0) 30 120/78

INFORMATION FOR THE PATIENT

You are Anita Savage, a 52-year-old woman. You have been married for twenty years, and live with your husband and two sons.

You are a computer programmer, work forty hours a week and sometimes work overtime to 52 hours.

You have been having pain over the right wrist for two months. You have tried paracetamol and Nurofen which has not helped. The pain is now affecting your job and you would like it to be sorted.

Information to reveal if asked

General information about yourself:

- You are a computer programmer working in an international computer firm. You have been working long hours lately and work eight hours a day or more till late evening. You constantly use the mouse and the keyboard.

- It is hard work but you do the extra work to pay for your sons' private school fees. You feel that these shifts leave you with very little time for relaxation and have been making you feel very tired. You attribute this to your age catching up.

- Your husband is supportive and there is no stress whatsoever on the home front. You plan to slow down in the next few years when the boys finish school.

- You had your last period two years ago and you are not experiencing any menopausal symptoms, such as flushing or mood swings.

Further details about your condition:

- You have pain in the right wrist. It is like a dull ache with numbness and tingling over the right thumb and index finger. You are right-handed.

- You have been working long hours lately and work eight hours a day or more till late evening.

- You don't have any low mood. You sleep a lot and wish you had more energy. You have very little time for relaxation. You have no time or energy for your hobbies like cross stich or knitting, or for exercise.

- You do not think you have lost weight, and you have no loss of appetite. In fact you have gained weight – a stone in the last six months since you stopped going to the gym.

- You do not have polyuria or polydipsia. You do suffer from constipation but have no other medical problems. You think your skin has got very dry and your hair is thinning. You think this is age-related.

Your ideas:

- You think you are getting old and do not have the energy you had a few years ago. You think your wrist problem could be due to constant use of the computer.

Your concerns:

- You don't want this wrist pain to affect your work.

Your expectations:

- You have tried painkillers. You want to try a splint. Your neighbour had wrist pain which settled with Nurofen and using a splint.

Information to reveal if examined

Phalen's sign positive

Tinel's sign positive

(see www.youtube.com/watch?v=Ze9piW3wgYw)

SUGGESTED APPROACH TO THE CONSULTATION

Targeted history taking:

- Obtain details on symptoms, progression, any trauma.
- Ask about patient's job, activities, hobbies, exercise, etc.
- Find out about symptoms related to weight, bowel habit, thirst, cardiac problems.
- Obtain a family history of CTS (there seems to be a strong genetic predisposition to CTS).

Clinical management:

- Discuss blood tests and diagnosis of CTS with hypothyroidism.
- Discuss treatment option for CTS; surgical and non-surgical interventions.
- Offer medications for patient's condition and arrange future blood tests and follow-ups.
- Fulfil her expectations of a wrist splint (wearing the splint to maintain the wrist in a neutral position for 12 hours daily, without compressing at the wrist, helps 50% of patients. Stop using the splint if there is no improvement by 12 weeks).

Interpersonal skills:

Good communication with the patient:

- discusses both diagnoses in a language the patient can understand.
- checks understanding and offers treatment options and follow-up plans.

BACKGROUND KNOWLEDGE REQUIRED FOR THIS CASE

CTS is the commonest peripheral nerve problem in the UK. Incidence peaks in late fifties, particularly in females. Obesity is a risk factor in younger patients. It is also common transiently in late pregnancy.

CTS may be the presenting symptom of an underlying disease such as diabetes mellitus, hypothyroidism or connective tissue disease (although additional tests seem to be of little value in typical CTS cases).

Standard symptoms

Dull aching discomfort in hand, forearm or upper arm

Paraesthesia in the hand

Weakness or clumsiness of the hand

Dry skin, swelling or colour changes in the hand

Occurrence of any of the above in the median nerve distribution

Provocation of symptoms in sleep

Provocation of symptoms by sustained hand or arm positions

Mitigation of symptoms by changing hand posture or shaking the wrist

Conditions that may be confused with CTS

Cervical radiculopathy (especially C6/7)

Ulnar neuropathy

Raynaud's phenomenon

Vibration white finger

Osteoarthritis of metacarpophalyngeal joint of the thumb

Tendonitis

Motor neuron disease

Syringomyelia

Multiple sclerosis

Treatments

Splinting

Steroids: local injection, local iontophoresis. Oral steroids could be helpful, but adverse effects tend to preclude their use. Refer for a steroid injection if symptoms are severe or if neurology is present or if a trial of conservation management over 3 months fails.

Surgical decompression

Management of subclinical hypothyroidism (NICE CKS, February 2011)

(see http://cks.nice.org.uk/hypothyroidism#!scenario:1)

How should I manage someone with subclinical hypothyroidism who has a thyroid-stimulating hormone (TSH) level of 10 mU/L or less?

- Confirm by repeat testing of thyroid stimulating hormone (TSH) and free thyroxine (FT_4) levels, with the addition of measurement of thyroid peroxidase antibodies (TPO-Ab), 3–6 months after the original result

- Levothyroxine treatment is not routinely recommended

- Consider offering levothyroxine treatment if:
  - the person has a goitre
  - their TSH level is rising
  - the woman is pregnant or planning pregnancy.

- Consider offering a trial of treatment if the person has symptoms compatible with hypothyroidism

- ○ prescribe treatment for a sufficient length of time to be able to judge whether there is symptomatic benefit
- ○ only continue treatment if there is a clear improvement in symptoms
- ○ if treatment is continued, once stable, measure TSH annually and alter the levothyroxine dose to maintain the TSH level within the reference range.

- If treatment is not offered, it is still necessary to monitor thyroid function to detect progression to overt hypothyroidism
  - ○ if the person has serum TPO-Abs, measure serum TSH and FT_4 annually, or earlier if symptoms develop
  - ○ otherwise, measure serum TSH and FT_4 approximately every 3 years, or earlier if symptoms develop.

Relevant literature

Bland, J (2007) **Carpal tunnel syndrome.** *BMJ*, **335**: 343.

de Rijk, MC, *et al.* (2007) **Does a carpal tunnel syndrome predict underlying disease?** *J. Neurol. Neurosurg. Psychiatry*, **78**: 635–637, doi:10 1136/jnnp. 2006.102145.

CASE 43 Palliative care (lung cancer)

INFORMATION FOR THE DOCTOR

This is a third party consultation with a district nurse.

Name	John Smith
Age	62
Social and family history	Lives with wife, retired accountant
Medical history	• Squamous cell carcinoma of bronchus with bone metastasis • On palliative register. Teams involved: district nurses, Macmillan team
Current medication	• Zomorph 80mg BD • Gabapentin 300mg TDS • Oromorph 5–10ml PRN • Lactulose 15ml BD • Ramipril 5mg OD • Simvastatin 40mg Nocte
Blood tests U&E	*Blood tests done yesterday* normal Sodium 136mmol/L (135–145) Potassium 3.3mmol/L (3.2–5) Urea 8.0mmol/L (1.7–8) Creatinine 86mmol/L (44–80)
FBC	normal Hb 13.2 WBC 7.0 Neutrophil 2.0 Plt 330
Serum calcium Corrected calcium	3.2mmol/L (2.1–2.5) 3.0mmol/L (2.1–2.5)
LFTs	normal
Urine	*Urine dipstix done this morning* negative for nitrites, leucocytes
BM	5.1

INFORMATION FOR THE PATIENT

You are district nurse Louise Glen, working with various teams looking after Mr John Smith. Mr Smith is reaching the end of his life. He is on the palliative register. He is a 62-year-old man with lung cancer. He has bony metastasis and is being cared for at home. The Macmillan palliative team is involved in his care.

Information to reveal if asked

General information about the patient:

- Mr Smith has battled with lung cancer for the last 3 years. He has squamous cell carcinoma of the bronchus. He has had extensive chemotherapy and radiotherapy for his condition but unfortunately this did not halt the progress of the disease. He now has bony metastasis with involvement of his spine and pelvis. He is being cared for at home.

- Mr Smith lives in his ground floor flat with his wife. The couple have no children but Mr Smith is very close to his nephew, who lives in London.

- He has always made his wishes clear and wishes to die in his own bed. He will want all his end-stage care to be commenced at home. He is not a practising Christian and does not have any religious requirements. He has made his will and all legal formalities are sorted. His nephew has been informed and will visit him later in the day.

Further details about Mr Smith's condition:

- He was coping very well until the last few weeks when his mobility gradually decreased due to pain in his legs and lower back. He has advanced metastatic disease but the pain was well controlled by opiates. He would usually spend his days in bed and armchair, reading or watching TV.

- DNs attend on a weekly basis for any minor problems like constipation, etc. Wife is aware of the situation.

- In the last two days, the patient seems to have increased lethargy and has got very confused. He is now completely bedbound. He seems very sleepy and is not himself. He is not in any respiratory distress or pain.

- Patient is not constipated, passed a bowel motion this morning, urine output has been good.

Your ideas:

- You feel that he is now end-stage and needs more input from the palliative team. You have spoken to the Macmillan team and they are happy to give their input. Mr Smith has deteriorated over the weekend and it is time to consider a syringe driver. You would like the GP to arrange for prescriptions for the driver.

Your concerns:

- You have no particular concerns but the symptoms you are worried about are the confusion and pain.

- You are worried that the confusion and pain imply that his condition has deteriorated. Should end of life care pathways be initiated?

Your expectations:

- You would like to set up a syringe driver and prescription for drugs. You have examined the patient, have sent some bloods and will be happy for a GP review if needed. You have the charts and would appreciate if they can be filled and signed for the syringe driver (mainly pain control: diamorphine and midazolam for confusion/restlessness).

Information to reveal if examined

BP 128/78, RR 18/min

P76 regular

PO_2 98% in air

Temp 36.2°C

Urine dip negative

SUGGESTED APPROACH TO THE CONSULTATION

Targeted history taking:

- Take a detailed medical and social history of the patient.

- Obtain details about his condition, progress and management plans.

- Take a social history, to include involvement of family or friends in his care, his spiritual beliefs and wishes.

- Get details of his symptoms, medications and any recent issues in his care.

- What are the patient's and family's wishes? Does Mr Smith have a living will?

Clinical management:

- Arrange an urgent home visit to review patient.

- Discuss blood results with the nurse and highlight the abnormalities and the need to treat them.

- Consider the hypercalcaemia. Should this be treated or not? Could it be treated at home? How do the family feel about treatment in a hospice?

- Mr Smith has advanced cancer and has expressed a desire to die at home. How distressing are his symptoms (bone pain, drowsiness, confusion and lethargy)? Does he need treatment with IV fluids or bisphosphonates or both? Can this treatment be delivered at home (perhaps by the district nurses, Macmillan team or outreach hospice team) or does it require admission to a hospice? If treatment is given, arrange for follow-up serum calcium checks.

- Discuss the blood results with the nurse. Based on Mr Smith's recent blood results, he has symptomatic hypercalcaemia. Whether to treat this or not depends on the wishes of the patient and his family and whether or not he is experiencing distressing or unpleasant symptoms.

- Discuss with the nurse whether or not she is happy to have this conversation with the family, who may have further questions about what the treatment for hypercalcaemia involves. She may want you to arrange the home visit and take this further.

Interpersonal skills:

Good communication with the district nurse:

- gathers information and discusses blood results.

- discusses treatment options for Mr Smith's condition and explains that treatable causes need to be looked into.

- takes into account the clinical limitations of another team member without being condescending or judgemental.

This case assesses the candidate's communication with team members and shared decision-making around end of life issues. The doctor's ability to respect the patient's autonomy, provide information about treatment options, offer the patient choice, and behave respectfully, is tested.

BACKGROUND KNOWLEDGE REQUIRED FOR THIS CASE

Management of person with hypercalcaemia who has known malignancy (NICE, CKS, December 2014)

(see http://cks.nice.org.uk/hypercalcaemia#!scenario:2)

How should I manage a person with hypercalcaemia who has a known malignancy?

- Consider whether it is appropriate to treat the hypercalcaemia
  - treatment of hypercalcaemia may not be appropriate if the person is receiving care for the last days of life.
- If the person has symptomatic hypercalcaemia, or moderate or severe hypercalcaemia (adjusted serum calcium concentration greater than 3.0mmol/L), admit immediately to hospital or a hospice if appropriate (preferably involving the person's specialist)
  - most people are managed with intravenous fluids and bisphosphonates (for example pamidronate)
- If the person has asymptomatic, mild hypercalcaemia (adjusted serum calcium concentration 3.0mmol/L or less), seek specialist advice about whether admission is needed and appropriate
  - while awaiting specialist advice:
    - advise about maintaining good hydration (drinking 3–4L of fluid per day), provided there are no contraindications (such as severe renal impairment or heart failure)
    - reassure that a low calcium diet is not necessary, as intestinal absorption of calcium is usually reduced
    - advise the person to avoid any drugs or vitamin supplements that could exacerbate the hypercalcaemia
    - encourage mobilisation where possible to avoid exacerbating the hypercalcaemia
    - advise the person to report any symptoms of hypercalcaemia.
- The frequency of monitoring of serum calcium following treatment will usually be specified by the specialist. Without treatment of the underlying cancer, hypercalcaemia usually returns 2–4 weeks after calcium-lowering treatment, and so calcium levels should be rechecked then if appropriate.

Topics for discussion

Reversible causes of confusion

Drugs: cimetidine, steroids, opioids, benzodiazepines, digoxin, lithium

Biochemical: hyponatraemia, hypercalcaemia, hypo- or hyperglycaemia

Drug/alcohol withdrawal

Infection, constipation, urinary retention, pain, hypoxia, anxiety, psychosocial distress.

Hypercalcaemia

Symptoms include drowsiness, confusion, nausea, vomiting, thirst, polyuria, weakness and constipation.

Management:

Fluid replacement

Bisphosphonates (zoledronic acid disodium, pamidronate, sodium clodronate)

Relevant literature

Adult Palliative Care Guideline Second Edition 2006, pp. 120 and 176

CASE 44 Obesity

INFORMATION FOR THE DOCTOR

Name	Beth Barraball
Age	28
Social and family history	• Non-smoker • Alcohol 4 units/week • Occupation: receptionist
Current medication	None
Blood tests TFTs Fasting blood glucose Cholesterol Plasma LDL Plasma triglyceride	*Blood tests done recently* normal 4.0 5.8 (2.8–5.0) 3.2mmol/L (0–3.0) 1.7mmol/L (0.8–1.7)

INFORMATION FOR THE PATIENT

You are Beth Barraball, a 22-year-old female. You work as a receptionist for a dentist. You don't smoke and are a social drinker. You are overweight, and have always been so.

You have a desk job. You work eight hours a day and longer hours on Wednesday when the practice is open for emergency appointments.

You have never been a healthy eater; you love junk food and desserts.

Your opening statement is *"Doctor I want to lose weight. Can I have a prescription for Alli?".*

Information to reveal if asked

Further information about yourself:

- You have always been overweight, a UK size 22–24. You have never seriously tried to lose weight. Your sister and mother have been big girls, so it runs in the family.

- You admit to eating junk food and have a sweet tooth. You love ice creams and frozen desserts.

- You are in a new relationship. Your boyfriend of two months has just proposed marriage and you plan to set a date for ten months' time.

- Your dietary routine is as follows: you have a heavy breakfast, then lunch at local fish and chip shop. Dinners are always takeaways from a local Balti joint.

- The only exercise you get is the short walk to the shopping centre during your lunch break. Evenings are spent in front of the TV or with Greg, your new boyfriend.

- You have tried diets like Slimming World and Atkins. You could not cope with the Atkins diet for more than a week as you love your potatoes.

- Your family history is as follows: your mother is on cholesterol tablets. Your sister is a big girl but is healthy, with no medical problems. Your father is well.

Your ideas:

- You know being overweight runs in the family as all the women are above size 20.

- Some of your friends have tried 'water tablets'. You have read on the internet that thyroid hormones can have an effect on slimming down or losing weight.

- You have heard of stomach banding and surgical options but will not want to consider something like it.

Your concerns:

- You want to slim down before the wedding. Greg is very tall and lanky and you appear to be huge in front of him. You want to drop a few pounds and look nicer for your wedding.

Your expectations:

- You would like to know about options of water tablets or thyroid hormones.

Medical history

You are fit and well, and not on any medications. You use condoms; you don't like any hormonal contraception as it affects your mood.

You have regular periods, 34 day cycle, bleed for 4 days. You don't think your periods are particularly heavy.

Information to reveal if examined

BP 120/76

Height 1.75m

Weight 92kg

BMI 30.0 (waist circumference 44 inches)

CVS NAD

RS NAD

SUGGESTED APPROACH TO THE CONSULTATION

Targeted history taking:

- Obtain details of weight gain, pattern and duration of symptoms, snoring and symptoms related to diabetes, hypothyroidism, Cushing's, PCOS, hypothalamic damage.

- Take a detailed dietary history, and one related to activity or exercise.

- Is there a family history of weight problems and related conditions like high cholesterol, cardiac problems, hypertension, strokes, etc.?

- Get details about socioeconomic status, such as income bracket.

- Take a history of medications which may aggravate weight gain.

Targeted examination:

- Weight, BMI, waist circumference, BP, cardiovascular and respiratory examination.

Clinical management:

- Use Motivational Interviewing style questions to discuss what changes the patient is willing to make to their usual eating and exercise habits.

- Encourage realistic goal-setting to achieve nutritionally-balanced, healthy eating and exercise approaching the recommended 30 min of moderate exercise per day, 5 days per week. Is the patient willing to consider an exercise referral scheme?

- Support the advice with appropriate written information (see *Relevant literature*).

- Offer options of referral to dietician.

- Discuss medications such as Orlistat, its side-effects and limitations.

- Clarify patient's ideas and notions in relation to water tablets/thyroid hormone pills.

Interpersonal skills:

Good communication with the patient:

- gives information about diuretics and thyroid hormones, clarifying that they have no role in treatment of obesity.

- discusses acceptable lifestyle options for losing weight.

- is realistic about patient's limitations.

- checks patient's understanding.

This case tests the doctor's ability to assess a common lifestyle problem that is likely to adversely affect the patient's long-term health. Some doctors could take the opportunity to scaremonger; others could be critical or dismissive or patronising. The aim is to educate and deliver appropriate behavioural intervention that produces long-lasting change.

First, it is important to get a good understanding of the problem through systematic data-gathering (obesity, level of risk, co-morbidity and potential health benefits from weight loss).

An effective communicator is able to build a supportive relationship with the patient through which goals are set and the patient motivated to make small and incremental changes. Some doctors like to use the structured approach from Motivational Interviewing to achieve a non-judgemental and holistic lifestyle intervention.

BACKGROUND KNOWLEDGE REQUIRED FOR THIS CASE

NICE (2014) guidelines (CG189) for Orlistat on obesity

Only prescribe Orlistat as part of an overall plan for managing obesity in adults who meet one of the following criteria:

- a BMI of 28kg/m^2 or more with associated risk factors
- a BMI of 30kg/m^2 or more.

Therapy should only continue for more than three months if the patient has lost at least 5% of their body weight from the drug treatment and similarly it should only continue for more than six months if weight loss has been at least 10% of body weight.

Make the decision to use drug treatment for longer than 12 months (usually for weight maintenance) after discussing potential benefits and limitations with the person. Treatment should not usually continue beyond 12 months and never beyond 24 months.

The co-prescribing of Orlistat with other drugs aimed at weight reduction is not recommended.

Orlistat (BNF, Sept 2014–March 2015)

Orlistat should be used in conjunction with other lifestyle measures to manage obesity; treatment should only be continued beyond 12 months after discussing potential benefits and risks with patient. Side-effects include oily leakage from rectum, flatulence, faecal urgency, faecal incontinence, abdominal distension and pain.

Relevant literature

Department of Health (2006) Your health, your weight. Available at: www.sheffieldachesandpains.com/assets/info%20leaflets/why%20weight%20matters.pdf

British Heart Foundation A guide to losing weight for men and women. Available at:

http://webarchive.nationalarchives.gov.uk/20130107105354/http://www.dh.gov.uk/prod_consum_dh/groups/dh_digitalassets/documents/digitalasset/dh_078132.pdf

http://bjgp.org/content/56/531/768

www.bradfordvts.co.uk/online-resources/0200-consultation/changing-behaviour/

CASE 45 Warts

INFORMATION FOR THE DOCTOR

Name	Daniel Fisher
Age	32
Social and family history	• Occupation: salesman (retail) • Smoker (10 cigarettes/day), alcohol (20 units/week) • Lives with his partner

Summary of consultation with GP colleague 2 weeks ago

"Presents with multiple skin lesions, mainly on face and trunk; asymptomatic but patient thinks they are unsightly. Also c/o intermittent tiredness. No symptoms of diabetes. No unexplained weight loss or night sweats. In stable same-sex relationship and thinking of getting married/applying for mortgage. Not had STI screening at onset of relationship.
Plan: Get FBC/HIV/Hep B serology and review with results."

Blood tests	Blood tests done 2 weeks ago	
FBC	Hb	12g/dL (13.5–18)
	Platelets	150×10^9/L (150–400)
	WBC	4×10^9/L (4–11)
	Neutrophils	1.5×10^9/L (2–7.5)
	Lymphocytes	0.8×10^9/L (1–4.5)
	Monocytes	0.8×10^9/L (0.2–0.8)
	Eosinophils	0.8×10^9/L (0.04–0.4)
	Basophil	0.1×10^9/L (<0.1)
Virology results	HIV positive (HIV 1 antibody detected)	
	Hepatitis B results negative	

INFORMATION FOR THE PATIENT

You are Daniel Fisher, a 32-year-old man. You work in a phone shop. You live with your partner. You have some warts on your body; recently you saw another GP colleague in the surgery for the warts who advised some blood tests, offered as screening. You are back to discuss these warts and see if the blood test results are back.

Your opening statement is *"Doctor, I had some blood tests done last week. I've had these warts and the other doctor suggested some tests".*

Shows photo (molluscum contagiosum, below). Multiple umbilicated lesions on trunk, thighs and face.

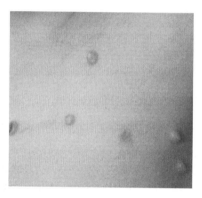

Image reproduced from http://scienceblogs.com

Information to reveal if asked

General information about yourself:

- You are a young gay man in a stable relationship.

- You live with your partner Tom Egerton, aged 30 years. You live in a rented flat. Tom is a jazz musician and both of you are doing well. You met Tom 3 years ago at a jazz festival and have been close since.

- You are well in yourself. You occasionally feel tired but attribute it to your busy job which involves travelling. You eat healthily, go to the gym three times a week and are trying to cut down on your smoking. Tom is a great cook and all your food is home-cooked; you eat a Mediterranean diet with plenty of fruit and vegetables.

- You and Tom are planning to get married next year and will be buying a house in London. Life seems very settled.

- You have been with your partner for three years but have had one-night stands with gay men before meeting Tom.

- You have never used IV drugs/recreational drugs. You and Tom don't use condoms; you have oral and anorectal sex.

Further details about your condition:

- You have noticed these warts over the last 8 months. It started as a single one on your upper lip and they are now coming up in crops in the last 2 months. They are all over your chest, thighs and a few over your face.

- Your partner Tom also has some on his abdomen.

Your ideas:

- You think one of you has caught it off the other. It could be related to swimming pool infection. You had been on a holiday to Tunisia 7 months ago. The hotel swimming pool was not up to your standards and you think you must have got something by swimming in there.

Your concerns:

- They seem to be spreading rapidly. The lesions on your face look unsightly. You are getting married next year and don't want all these warts on your face or body.

Your expectations:

- You want to get rid of the warts. Tom will be seeing his own GP for the same problem. He is registered at another surgery and is happy to undergo any tests and get treated for it.

- You agreed to get tested for HIV and hepatitis B. This was suggested by your GP colleague when you saw him last week and a sample was taken by the nurse the same day. In fact this had crossed your mind when Tom proposed marriage last year and you are now planning to buy a house. You are here for the test results and want to know any possible treatments for the warts.

Social history

You have had several male partners in the past. You admit to having one-night stands with unknown men while visiting gay festivals and parades in foreign countries. You love Berlin and visited the city every year for six years before meeting Tom; you attended the Christopher Street Day festivities in Berlin and enjoyed it very much. You had unprotected oral and anal sex with unknown men at the festival.

SUGGESTED APPROACH TO THE CONSULTATION

Targeted history taking:

- Obtain details about the skin lesions, treatment tried and progression.
- Take a detailed sexual history.
- Are there any other ongoing medical problems, or health deterioration?
- What symptoms are causing distress? Are there any particular concerns about the lesions?

Targeted examination:

- An examination is not required.

Clinical management:

- Address patient's concerns and ideas about the possible reasons for the warts.
- Break bad news that he is HIV positive and offer referral to HIV clinic for HIV medications.
- Highlight the importance of partner being tested for HIV.
- Arrange referral to HIV clinic as per local protocols.
- Arrange follow-up so that the patient can present with questions he may think about after being given today's results. It also gives him an opportunity to present with his partner, if either so wishes.
- One of the options for molluscum contagiosum would be waiting and watching.
- Other treatment options would be cryotherapy or referral to skin clinic for topical creams or laser treatment.

Interpersonal skills:

This case tests the doctor's ability to discuss an unwelcome test result and deal with the patient's subsequent distress and queries. It is important to have a structure in this case so that the doctor is able to deal with all the tasks of the consultation in the time given.

Good communication with the patient:

- is sensitive and shows empathy to the nature of problem.
- is non-judgemental to presentation of sexual history.
- provides sufficient information to the patient to enable decision making.
- clarifies and corrects patient's concepts about warts and swimming pool.
- breaks bad news with sensitivity, offering hope and support.

BACKGROUND KNOWLEDGE REQUIRED FOR THIS CASE

Breaking bad news

The following model could be used to structure the communication with the patient: http://hiv.ubccpd.ca/files/2012/09/Summary-on-Breaking-Bad-News.pdf

Molluscum contagiosum

Molluscum contagiosum is a benign self-limiting viral infection caused by a DNA virus of the pox family.

This condition may occur in adults presenting to STD clinics where the disease has been transmitted during sexual contact and in immunodeficient patients (AIDS).

Most people do not require treatment, as lesions will usually resolve within 1–2 years, and do not limit activities or cause symptoms.

No treatments are licensed in the UK for treating molluscum contagiosum.

If lesions are troublesome or considered unsightly, use simple trauma or cryotherapy:

- Squeezing lesions (with fingernails) or piercing them (orange stick) may be tried, following a bath. Treatment should be limited to a few lesions at one time.
- Cryotherapy may be used in older children or adults, if the healthcare professional is experienced in the procedure.

The following treatments may be considered by a specialist:

- Surgical (e.g. curettage, cautery)
- Topical (e.g. pulsed dye laser, phenol ablation, imiquimod 5%, cantharidin, potassium hydroxide 10%, podophyllin, silver nitrate paste, benzoyl peroxide 10%, and retinoids).

Relevant literature

BASHH (2008) *United Kingdom National Guideline on the Management of Molluscum Contagiosum* (www.bashh.org/documents/26/26.pdf)

NICE CKS (Sept 2012)

Trurchin, I and Barankin, B (2006) **Dermacase.** *Can. Fam. Physician,* **52(11)**: 1395–1407.

CASE 46 Aches and pains

INFORMATION FOR THE DOCTOR

Name	Salma Sheikh
Age	32
Social and family history	• Married, non-smoker, teetotaller • Muslim housewife, lives with husband and two children aged 3 and 6
Medical history	• Epilepsy: controlled • Atopic dermatitis • Haemorrhoids
Current medication	• Carbamazapine 400mg BD • Diprobase ointment topical PRN • Proctosedyl ointment PRN
Blood tests Hb ESR WBC TSH T$_4$ U&E LFTs Glucose Vitamin D Calcium Corrected calcium Parathyroid hormone	*Blood tests done two weeks ago* 13.0g/dL 5mm/hour normal 3.6 (0.3–4.2) 13.3 (12.0–22.0) normal normal 4.6mmol/L (3.2–11.0) 17nmol/L (50–120) 1.72mmol/L (2.15–2.55) 1.98mmol/L (2.1–2.5) 62mg/L (15–65)

Consultation with your colleague Dr Agrawal 2 weeks ago:

(History and interpretation by Ms Najma Begum, friend of Ms Sheikh)

"Patient has been having bone pain and feeling tired for 6 months. Pains in both knees, hips and lower back. No red flags like weight loss, appetite loss or change in bowel habit. No red flags for back pain. No joint swelling. Examination shows normal movements at knees/hip joints. Back examination NAD.
Advised paracetamol/ ibuprofen as needed.
Referred for blood tests with follow-up appointment in 2 weeks."

INFORMATION FOR THE PATIENT

This is a follow-up appointment.

You are 32-year-old Salma Sheikh. You are a mother of two children, recently arrived in the UK. You live with your husband and children in a council flat.

You and your family are asylum seekers from Afghanistan. You arrived in the UK a year ago. You were granted asylum 7 months ago. Your family is on benefits. You live in a two-bedroom council flat.

You are a school drop-out and your husband was a carpenter in Kabul. You speak very limited English. Your husband has enrolled for English speaking classes and plans to look for work soon.

Your 6 year old daughter has started attending a local primary school and your son attends a nursery part-time. Your son's place in nursery, which he attends two mornings per week, is state-funded.

Information to reveal if asked

General information about yourself:

You are a housewife and manage the house and children. Your husband drops the children at school and nursery then attends his English classes. He is attending classes for spoken English four times a week. Fridays are for household chores and his religious commitments.

You attend the mosque for Friday prayers and occasionally go out shopping with your husband over the weekend.

You have managed this appointment, and the one two weeks ago when you had blood tests done, with great difficulty. Your friend has been kind enough to make time for you and accompany you to the GP both times.

Further details about your condition:

- You have been feeling very tired lately. You have been having generalised aches and pains with constant pain in your thighs and feet. You wake up in the morning with no energy and want to lie in bed all day.

- You came to see the doctor two weeks ago with tiredness and pain in your bones. The doctor did blood tests and asked you to return in 2 weeks.

- You live on the fourth floor of the building and the lift has been non-functional for three months. Climbing up the stairs leaves you exhausted and you have stopped going to the mosque. You have not been out for nearly three months except for occasional Sunday trips to a local open market. Ali, your husband, does all the chores.

- You do not have weight or appetite loss. There is no polyuria or polydipsia. There is no change in your bowel habit. You do not report any recent weight gain either and there is no cold intolerance.

- You have regular periods with no symptoms of menorrhagia. You have a 26-day cycle and bleed for 3 days.

- You almost confined to your flat due to lack of social support. You speak Pashtu and there are very few Afghani women around. Language barriers and health issues add to your difficulties in getting around. You have a friend, Fauzia who you met at the mosque 6 months ago. She visits you once a month as she lives far away and needs to take two buses to get to your address.

- You don't have many hobbies. You once enjoyed needlework and sewing but have no equipment or scope to pursue it in the UK.

- You deny being in low mood. Your appetite is normal and you sleep a lot as you feel tired and 'achey' all the time. You have had no self-harming thoughts.

Your ideas:

- Your grandmother also had aching joints all her life and you think this could be a family problem. She never had any formal diagnosis and did not see a doctor for it.

Your concerns:

- You see yourself as a traditional Muslim housewife spending her time around the household and children. You are not particularly bothered about the social isolation. Your priorities are your husband and children. You are worried that you may not be able to fulfil all your duties.

Your expectations:

- You want to feel better. You want relief from these constant aches and pains so that you are able to cope with your daily chores.

Medical history

You have well-controlled epilepsy. You have been seizure-free for 12 years and started on medications 14 years ago in Kabul. You also use emollients for skin problems. You occasionally have had rectal bleeds but that is not an issue any more.

Social history

You have hardly any friends and are socially isolated. You are a traditional Muslim lady and wear the hijab. You fast for Ramadan and your dietary requirements include halal meat.

Information to reveal if examined

BMI 22

Blood pressure normal

Cardiovascular examination normal

Musculoskeletal findings NAD

SUGGESTED APPROACH TO THE CONSULTATION

Targeted history taking:

- Take a detailed history of symptoms, any joint swelling, joint pains, symptoms related to tiredness to include thyroid problems, diabetes. Red flags to be ruled out.

- Obtain details about medications.

- Ask about diet, exercise and exposure to sunlight.

Targeted examination:

Baseline BP, cardiovascular examination.

Clinical management:

- Interpret the blood results: Vitamin D is 17nmol/L, which indicates deficiency. Explain vitamin D deficiency, its possible causes and its treatment to the patient. Provide information in a way the patient is able to understand and check her understanding at regular intervals.

- If she has difficulty understanding the information, offer to provide written information or arrange follow-up with an interpreter.

- Offer high dose oral vitamin D, as 50 000IU capsule once weekly for 6w, or 20 000IU capsule two per week for 7w, or 800IU capsules five per day for 10w.

- Arrange follow-up, to check for corrected calcium in a month and to start maintenance therapy.

Interpersonal skills:

Good communication with patient:

- understands limitations and difficulties in relation to language barriers.

- understands socioeconomic and cultural barriers which may limit treatment.

- shows empathy and works towards a shared goal.

BACKGROUND KNOWLEDGE REQUIRED FOR THIS CASE

Vitamin D deficiency

Vitamin D deficiency is common in the UK population. Risk factors include skin pigmentation, use of sunscreen or concealing clothing, being elderly or institutionalised, obesity, malabsorption, renal or liver disease and anticonvulsant use.

Adults present with pain and proximal muscle weakness. Rib, hip, pelvis, thigh and foot pain are typical. More diffuse muscular aches and muscle weakness, including in limbs and back, are common.

UK Department of Health recommendations

All pregnant and breastfeeding women should take a daily supplement containing 10mcg of vitamin D.

All infants and young children aged 6 months to 5 years should take a daily supplement containing vitamin D in vitamin drops to meet requirement of 7–8.5mcg of vitamin D per day. (However, infants receiving fortified formula will not need additional drops.)

People aged 65 years and over and people who are not exposed to much sun should also take a daily supplement containing 10mcg of vitamin D.

Healthy Start Scheme

www.healthystart.nhs.uk

A UK government-run scheme, where patients can get free vouchers every week which they can swap for milk, fresh fruit, fresh vegetables and infant formula milk.

Patients are eligible for free vitamins if on Jobseekers Allowance, pregnant, under 18, receiving income support or child tax credit.

Relevant literature

Department of Health letter (2012) **Vitamin D – advice on supplements for at risk groups.** Reference cem/cmo/2012/04.

Pearce, SH and Cheetham, TD (2010) **Diagnosis and management of Vitamin D deficiency.** *BMJ*, 340:b5664. doi: 10.1136/bmj.b5664.
Available at: www.bmj.com/content/340/bmj.b5664.

CASE 47 LUTS/Urinary symptoms

INFORMATION FOR THE DOCTOR

Name	Albert Elwood
Age	82
Social and family history	Ex-smoker (last smoked 40 years ago), teetotaller
Medical history	• BPH (benign prostatic hypertrophy) for 7 years • Hypothyroidism • Osteoarthritis • Depression
Current medication	• Levothyroxine 50mcg OD • Adcal D3 tablets BD • Citalopram 10mg OD • Doxazosin 4mg OD

INFORMATION FOR THE PATIENT

You are Albert Elwood, an 82-year-old widower. You live alone in a 3-bedroom bungalow and manage well. Your wife died 3 years ago, her loss left you bereaved and depressed but you are coping well with antidepressants. Your daughter lives away but visits you once a month.

You have had urinary symptoms for some years but these have recently worsened.

Information to reveal if asked

General information about yourself:

- You live alone, manage well, rarely see a doctor. You are here today because of worsening of your waterworks. You have had an enlarged prostate and have been on tablets for 7 years. Urinary symptoms are now affecting the quality of your life.

Further details about your condition:

- Lately there has been worsening of symptoms with urgency and straining. You also get a feeling of incomplete emptying.

- Nocturia is troublesome; you wake up 3–4 times a night which leaves you very tired. You have been getting aches and pains and a backache. You have lost appetite and weight lately.

- Your brother has prostate cancer but is stable and doing well. Your nephew and uncle have the disease as well.

Your ideas:

- You saw a urologist five years ago; you were told you might need an operation in the future but had postponed it. You were managing well then, your wife was alive and you did not take the option. You think that the prostate is big enough to warrant a surgical intervention.

Your concerns:

- Your symptoms leave you very tired and it is getting difficult to cope. You are worried about the surgery itself and how you would manage after the operation. Your daughter has four children, lives away and you have no help at home. You are also worried about complications of surgery and want to know how long you will have to stay in the hospital after a procedure.

Your expectations:

- You want to be re-referred to the specialist to look into your prostate problems and consider the operation.

Medical history

Benign prostatic hypertrophy for 7 years. Hypothyroidism with stable TFTs.

Information to reveal if examined

BP 128/68mmHg P77 regular

Abdomen – non-tender, no palpable masses. No inguinal nodes.

PR examination – hard fixed prostate.

SUGGESTED APPROACH TO THE CONSULTATION

Targeted history taking:

- Take a detailed history of LUTS: filling symptoms like urinary frequency, urgency, dysuria, nocturia. Obstructive symptoms like poor stream, hesitancy, dribbling, incomplete voiding and overflow incontinence.
- Obtain details on possible infective aetiology like symptoms of fever, loin pain/pelvic pain, haematuria, history of UTIs.
- Get a history of sexual and erectile dysfunction in age-appropriate patients.

Targeted examination:

- Examine the abdomen, including external genital examination and digital rectal examination.
- Examination should include blood pressure check, palpable nodes and a urine dipstick test.
- Men with bothersome LUTS to complete a urinary frequency volume chart and a validated symptoms chart, e.g. I-PSS (the International Prostate Symptom Score).

Clinical management:

- Discuss your clinical findings, especially the fixed hard irregular prostate on rectal examination and the back (bone) pain on history.
- Arrange for an urgent urinary dipstix, urine MC&S and a PSA.
- Tell the patient what you would like to do if his PSA comes back as raised for his age, i.e. your intention to refer him to urology on the two week wait. Check that he wants this investigation and referral.
- Arrange follow-up.

Interpersonal skills:

Good communication with the patient:

- is empathetic, gives information in a way the patient understands.
- breaks bad news about possibility of prostate cancer which will need further investigations and referrals.
- checks understanding and offers follow-up.

BACKGROUND KNOWLEDGE REQUIRED FOR THIS CASE

NICE CKS Prostate cancer (2011)

Primary care will be involved in shared care with follow-up and monitoring, and early recognition and initial management of the complications of the condition and adverse effects of its treatment.

- Treatments for localised prostate cancer
  - Treatment options include:
    - no active treatment: watchful waiting, and active surveillance.
    - radical treatment: radical prostatectomy, external beam radiotherapy, brachytherapy.
    - focal treatments: high intensity focused ultrasound and cryotherapy are used in clinical trials.
    - adjuvant treatment: hormonal treatment, including androgen blockade and androgen withdrawal—a short course may be given before or during radical radiotherapy.
- Treatments for locally advanced prostate cancer, metastatic prostate cancer, or relapse after radical treatment include:
  Neoadjuvant and concurrent luteinising hormone-releasing hormone agonist or antagonist therapy—see hormonal treatment.
  - Adjuvant hormonal treatment.
  - Radiotherapy: external beam radiotherapy and brachytherapy.
  - Prostatectomy: radical prostatectomy, high intensity focused ultrasound, and cryotherapy.
  - Chemotherapy—some centres may not provide some treatments, such as those being researched in clinical trials.

Prostate cancer

Referral guidelines for suspected cancer (NICE guidelines CG27, 2005)

The prostate is a small gland found only in men. Symptoms of prostate cancer include:

- difficulty passing urine
- a weak or sometimes intermittent flow of urine
- difficulty in starting to pass urine
- blood in the urine
- lower back pain
- bone pain
- weight loss, especially in older men
- erectile dysfunction (an inability to get or keep an erection firm enough for sexual activity).

Tests

Any patients with symptoms of prostate cancer should be given a digital rectal examination.

Request prostate-specific antigen (PSA). Before a PSA test exclude a urine infection using a urine dipstix or MSU for MC&S. Any infection should be treated and a PSA test delayed until 1 month after the infection has gone.

Urgent referral

An urgent referral should be made in patients with:

- a hard, irregular prostate (PSA levels should also be tested). If the prostate is simply enlarged and the PSA level is in the age-specific range an urgent referral is not needed
- PSA levels above the age-specific range, with or without lower urinary tract symptoms, and a normal prostate
- symptoms and high PSA levels.

In patients with a borderline level of PSA and no other symptoms of prostate cancer, the GP should carry out another PSA test 1 to 3 months later. If the second test shows that the PSA level is rising, the GP should refer the patient urgently.

CASE 48 Erectile dysfunction

INFORMATION FOR THE DOCTOR

Name	Paul Wills
Age	46
Social and family history	• Unemployed, lives with partner • Alcohol 10 units a week, occasional smoker
Medical history	Hypertension
Current medications	Ramipril 10mg.
Blood tests S testosterone Free testosterone S sex binding globulin Fasting glucose Total cholesterol LDL HDL Triglycerides	*Blood tests done recently* 4.5nmol/L (6.6–25.7) 98pmol/L (163–473) 38nmol/L (19.0–76.0) 6.9mmol/L (3.2–6.0) 6.8mmol/L (2.8–5.0) 3.8mmol/L (0–3.0) 1.3mmol/L (0.8–1.8) 2.3mmol/L (0.8–1.7)

Details of last consultation with Dr Banajee:

"At end of BP check/medication review patient mentions problems with erections. Advised to get some blood tests and book a separate consultation to discuss this in detail. Advised ED unlikely to be due to ramipril; meds issued. Health education – diet and exercise."

INFORMATION FOR THE PATIENT

You are Paul Wills, a 46-year-old man living with your partner. You are unemployed, and are currently looking for work. You have done various jobs like working in supermarkets, bookshops and retail. You were made redundant 6 months ago. Your last job was working on a deli counter.

Your opening statement is *"I have an embarrassing problem. I think I need to try Viagra"*.

Information to reveal if asked

Further details about yourself:

- You do not have any financial worries. Your partner has a steady job. She works in a nursery.

Further details about your condition:

- You have experienced loss of libido over six months and lately have been having difficulty in achieving and maintaining erections.

- You have been in a stable relationship for two years, you have a good relationship; you find your partner attractive but lately have been finding it difficult to maintain an erection. Your partner is very understanding.

- Your mood is stable and you are not depressed. Your appetite is good and in fact you have recently put on a lot of weight. You sleep well and still take pleasure in all the activities you were doing before. You love your DIY and do it on and off.

- You otherwise feel well in yourself, are on blood pressure tablets and your BP is well controlled.

- You do not have a personal or family history of heart problems or diabetes.

Your ideas:

- You have read on the internet that smoking and alcohol could be linked to this problem and are trying to cut down.

- You are not keen on counselling as you do not have a relationship problem. Both of you are happy with each other and there is no third person involved.

- You have read about Viagra and are keen to try it.

Your concerns:

- You don't have major concerns at the moment but think it could have an impact on the relationship in the long run and affect your sex life.

Your expectations:

- You want a prescription for Viagra.

- You are happy to do a blood test.

Information to reveal if examined

BMI 31

Genital examination normal

BP 130/78mmHg

SUGGESTED APPROACH TO THE CONSULTATION

Targeted history taking:

- Obtain details about patient's symptoms. This should include libido, erectile quality, frequency and quality of nocturnal erections, function on masturbation.

- Any weight gain, changes in pattern of body hair or any skin alteration?

- Family history of prostate problems, cardiovascular problems, strokes?

- Obtain personal details about relationships.

- Take a medical history to include any conditions which may be linked to erectile dysfunction; drug history.

- Enquire about recent mood, cognitive function, sleep pattern.

Clinical management:

- Address Paul's lifestyle issues, especially his high BMI and cholesterol, and discuss the link to metabolic syndrome.

- Could consider an endocrine review in view of his low testosterone.

- Look into symptom management with use of Viagra.

- Arrange follow-up to investigate hyperglycaemia by arranging further blood tests such as repeat testosterone (non-fasting), LH, FSH, prolactin, HBAc, TSH and LFTs.

Interpersonal skills:

Good communication with the patient:

- acknowledges the patient's agenda (to get treatment, preferably Viagra, for his erectile dysfunction). The good communicator is able to broaden the discussion into possible causes of ED and the patient's personal risk factors for ED, which require further investigation. The doctor gives information in simple language which the patient can understand, developing the patient's ideas and expectations.

- highlights the importance of making lifestyle changes and explains the link with metabolic syndrome, diabetes, and cardiovascular disease.

- checks understanding and reassures patient.

BACKGROUND KNOWLEDGE REQUIRED FOR THIS CASE

Late onset hypogonadism

- Late onset hypogonadism, sometimes called the male menopause, is defined as a "clinical and biochemical syndrome associated with advancing age and characterised by typical symptoms and a deficiency in serum testosterone levels".
- Symptoms of the andropause include reduced growth of secondary body hair, decrease in muscle mass, increased central body fat, loss of libido, erectile dysfunction, lethargy, reduced ability to concentrate and mood changes.
- It may significantly reduce quality of life and adversely affect the function of multiple organ systems.
- Complications of the andropause include osteoporosis, metabolic problems, increased heart disease and all-cause mortality, depression and cognitive decline.
- The prevalence of hypogonadism is higher in men with metabolic syndrome, type 2 diabetes, coronary heart disease, COPD, autoimmune disorders and HIV infection. Low testosterone concentrations are associated with several cardiovascular risk factors, including visceral obesity, insulin resistance, dyslipidaemia, hypertension and prothrombotic and pro-inflammatory states.
- Measurement of serum testosterone can be problematic due to hour-to-hour variations in testosterone level and binding of testosterone to SHBG. For example, testosterone levels may be low the morning after a man has consumed a large amount of alcohol or raised if the patient is fasting. Testosterone bound to SHBG is tightly bound and not usable by the body. SHBG levels increase by around 1% per year as men age.
- Treatment is with testosterone supplements once prostate cancer has been excluded (testosterone may exacerbate prostate cancer that is already present). In ageing men, there is some debate over when and how to treat primary hypogonadism and the effects of treatment. As a general principle, treatment should be considered if the potential benefit (treatment of symptoms/ reducing CV risk) exceeds the potential harm (risk of prostate cancer).

Relevant literature

Jones, TH (2009) **Late onset hypogonadism**. *BMJ*, **338**: 352.

CASE 49 Depression

INFORMATION FOR THE DOCTOR

Name	Nazneen Begum
Age	24
Social and family history	• Married, non-smoker, teetotaller • Occupation: housewife
Current medication	Sumatriptan PRN

INFORMATION FOR THE PATIENT

You are 24-year-old Nazneen Begum, a recently-married housewife.

You arrived in the UK six months ago from Bangladesh following an arranged marriage. Your husband works in the catering industry. You have no children.

You feel lonely; you have no friends or social circle. You miss your family in Dhaka. Your husband has been understanding, and tries to find time to build the relationship. You spend the entire day in your one-bedroom flat, occasionally going to the corner shop to buy essential groceries. Your husband works as a kitchen help till evening and sometimes at weekends. He takes you out when he gets time, which can be over the weekends. You call your family in Bangladesh every day but this is clearly not helping.

Your opening statement is *"I don't think I can cope any longer".*

Information to reveal if asked

General information about yourself:

- You have an IT degree and had worked in an IT firm prior to marriage.
- You have an arranged marriage. Ahmed is a distant cousin who was chosen by your parents.
- You do want to work as it makes you feel independent and confident. You haven't explored the job prospects in the UK. Ahmed is very encouraging about you having a career.

Further details about your condition:

- You feel low, and cry all the time when by yourself. Your appetite is low. You are taking no pleasure in dressing up or shopping. You are sleeping well.
- You have no self-harming thoughts and won't do anything like that as you love your parents and brothers very much.

Your ideas:

- You think you should never have married Ahmed but agreed to do so because of parental pressure. You have no interest in having sex with your husband and the sexual aspect of marriage is the main stressor.
- You think you have made a wrong decision and don't know how to get out of this situation.

Your concerns:

- You are confused about your sexual preference. You have never been in a relationship with a woman but were attracted to a colleague back home where she worked in an office. The attraction was mutual but it did not progress to a relationship as you got married and moved to the UK.

- Men have never turned you on. You are not keen on this marriage but will not take any decision before seeing a counsellor.

Your expectations:

- You have not told your husband yet and would like to be referred for counselling to help resolve these conflicts.

- You are happy to try medications while you await counselling.

Information to reveal if asked

PHQ-9 score 23

SUGGESTED APPROACH TO THE CONSULTATION

Targeted history taking:

- Take a detailed personal and social history.
- Assess what symptoms of depression the patient has, and how these impact on her functionally and socially. Assess the risk of suicide, by asking *"Do you ever think about suicide or imagine ending your life?"*
- Explore if there are any safeguarding concerns for children or vulnerable adults.
- Look for co-morbid conditions associated with depression including: alcohol or substance abuse; anxiety; eating disorders; psychotic symptoms and dementia.
- Obtain details about symptoms related to mood, sleep, appetite, anhedonia.
- Ask about use of alcohol and drugs, previous mental health problems, social support systems to access if feeling very low, especially when alone.
- Rule out presence of self-harming thoughts or suicidal ideation.

Targeted examination:

- Perform a PHQ-9. Questionnaires such as this can help identify people with depression and indicate severity. They should not be used as the sole method for diagnosing depression and for deciding on whether to offer treatment.
- Rule out psychosis.
- Assess risk of DSH and impulsivity.

Clinical management:

- Discuss guided self-help (such as Overcoming Depression books or computerised CBT); counselling; exercise; and discuss the option of medication. Consider giving the patient written information or directing them to a decision aid which they can access at home, with the option of returning in a few days with their decision.
- Offer information on organisations and groups or local network which may help patient to improve social contact.
- Discuss options of medications and inform about duration and side-effects of drugs.
- Arrange referral for counselling and arrange follow-up within 2 weeks.

Interpersonal skills:

Good communication with the patient:

- is empathetic, offers hope and support.
- offers options and provides information and guidance.

BACKGROUND KNOWLEDGE REQUIRED FOR THIS CASE

Key priorities for implementation of the NICE depression guidelines (CG90 and CG91)

- A comprehensive assessment of patients with possible depression should be carried out which does not rely on a simple symptom count, but takes into account the degree of functional impairment and/or disability.

- People with subthreshold symptoms, or mild to moderate depression, should be offered low-intensity psychosocial interventions, including guided self-help based on the principles of cognitive-behavioural therapy (CBT), computerised CBT, and/or a structured group physical activity programme.

- Antidepressant drug treatment should be considered for patients with subthreshold or mild depression where there is a past history of moderate or severe depression, and where subthreshold symptoms or mild depression have persisted for more than 2 years, or not responded to low-intensity psychosocial interventions. Citalopram or sertraline are suggested as the first choice of antidepressant.

- Psychological and psychosocial interventions should be based on manuals, and delivered by competent practitioners.

- Patients should be advised that antidepressants are not addictive and encouraged to continue medication for at least 6 months after remission.

- Cognitive-behavioural therapy should be offered to those who relapse or fail to recover with drug treatment alone.

- A combination of antidepressants and manualised psychological therapy (CBT or interpersonal therapy) should be offered to patients with moderate to severe depression.

- Mindfulness-based cognitive therapy to prevent relapse should be considered where there have been three or more previous episodes of depression.

From: Kendrick, T and Peveler, R (2010) Guidelines for the management of depression: NICE work? *Br. J. Psych.* 197 (5): 345–347; DOI: 10.1192/bjp. bp.109.074575

CASE 50 Testicular pain

INFORMATION FOR THE DOCTOR

Name	Kevin Graham
Age	26
Social and family history	• Occupation: manager at a food outlet • Lives with girlfriend • Non-smoker, alcohol 14 units/week

INFORMATION FOR THE PATIENT

You are Kevin Graham, a 26-year-old man. You are a manager at a Subway food outlet. You live with your girlfriend.

You are fit and well, have no medical problems and are not on any medications.

You have been having testicular pains for 5 days; these have now got worse. The pain is in both testicles. You think your testes are red but not particularly swollen. They have a dull ache and you have been able to go to work today. You took paracetamol which has not helped.

Information to reveal if asked

Further details about your condition:

- You have been feeling unwell, hot and sweaty last evening. There has been whitish penile discharge.

- You are fit and well, prone to occasional UTIs (had UTI as a teenager), no urine symptoms at present.

- You have been in a stable relationship with your girlfriend for 2 years but you had a 'one night stand' two weeks ago at a stag party with friends. This sexual encounter was 'paid for' by your friend who hosted the party.

- You did not use a condom. You have not had sex since as your girlfriend is away on a business trip.

Your ideas:

- You think this could be a sexual infection from the encounter you had at the stag party.

Your concerns:

- You are worried that you could have picked up a sexually transmitted infection and want to be treated. You do not want your girlfriend to know and do not want to pass on the infection.

Your expectations:

- You want to be treated for this problem.

Information to reveal if examined

On examination, both testicles red, tender. No hydrocele.

Temperature 38°C

SUGGESTED APPROACH TO THE CONSULTATION

Targeted history taking:

- Take a detailed sexual history, including details about known/unknown partners, use of barrier method/condom use and type of sexual encounter.
- Obtain a history of symptoms.
- Obtain vaccination history for mumps in cases of testicular swelling.

Clinical management:

- Discuss the most probable diagnosis (epididymo-orchitis).
- Discuss the most likely cause, i.e. an STI. Given the purulent penile discharge, the causative organism is likely to be *N. gonorrhoeae*.
- Discuss the option of testing for STIs, either by GP or at an STI clinic. If the patient opts for testing in GP practice, explain how the urine specimen is collected and how he will be informed of the results.
- As *N. gonorrhoeae* is developing drug resistance, discuss the need for IM antibiotics and discuss whether the practice is able to administer IM ceftriaxone. Current treatment for gonorrhoea is with a single IM injection of ceftriaxone (500mg) combined with a single dose of oral azithromycin (1g).
- Discuss review in 2 weeks after treatment to obtain a repeat test to ensure eradication of the infection. The patient should be advised to avoid sex until 48 hours after both they and their partner have been treated. Discuss the need for contact tracing; GUM clinic has the skills and resources for this.

Interpersonal skills:

Good communication with the patient:

- explores the symptoms and is empathetic to the patient's discomfort. Discusses the diagnosis and management in a way the patient can understand.
- is non-judgemental and reassures regarding confidentiality.

BACKGROUND KNOWLEDGE REQUIRED FOR THIS CASE

Gonorrhoea

Most men with gonorrhoea present with symptoms of dysuria and penile discharge, which is usually profuse and purulent. These symptoms typically develop fairly rapidly (2–5 days) after sexual contact with an infected partner.

Women can also have symptoms of discharge, but most infections in females remain asymptomatic and are only diagnosed when microbiology testing is carried out.

Advances in molecular methods have improved the detection of gonorrhoea because these methods are more tolerant to delays in transport to the laboratory and can be used with specimens, such as urine or self-taken vaginal swabs, allowing more patients to be screened both in primary care settings and specialised clinics.

If left untreated, gonorrhoea can spread locally and, rarely, develop systemically.

Men may develop epididymo-orchitis, with swelling and tenderness in the scrotum developing over a period of 12–24 hours. More uncommonly, a para-urethral abscess or sinus can develop.

The main concern in women is salpingitis, with subsequent tubal damage leading to infertility, chronic pain or future ectopic pregnancy. The risk of tubal damage is, however, lower with gonorrhoea than with chlamydia.

Current treatment for gonorrhoea is with a single IM injection of ceftriaxone (500mg) combined with a single dose of oral azithromycin (1g).

Oral cefixime (single dose 400mg) is not recommended as first-line treatment, owing to the lower tissue levels achieved with oral dosing. It should only be used if no alternative treatment is available and referral to a sexual health clinic is not possible. A repeat test is recommended two weeks after treatment to ensure eradication of the infection.

The patient should be advised to avoid sex until 48 hours after both they and their partner have been treated, and tracing, screening and empirical treatment of their partner is therefore recommended.

If the index patient is symptomatic, all partners from within the past two weeks should be seen (or their last partner if this was longer ago).

Patients who have gonorrhoea are at an increased risk of acquiring it again in future and their initial presentation offers an opportunity to provide advice on safer sex. Cole, M, Ross, J and Ison, C (2013) Sexual health – antimicrobial resistant gonorrhoea. GPonline.com

Epididymo-orchitis

Acute epididymo-orchitis is a clinical syndrome consisting of pain, swelling and inflammation of epididymis +/– testes. The most common route of infection is local extension and is mainly due to infections spreading from urethra (STI) or bladder (urinary pathogens).

Aetiology

Under 35: most often *Chlamydia trachomatis* and *N. gonorrhoeae*.

Over 35: most often non-sexually transmitted Gram-negative enteric organisms causing UTI.

Men who engage in insertive anal intercourse are at risk of sexually transmitted enteric organisms.

Mumps should be considered as an aetiology.

Differential diagnosis

Testicular torsion. A painful swollen testicle in an adolescent or young man should be managed as torsion unless proven otherwise.

Treatment

Recommended regimens:

1. For epididymo-orchitis due to any sexually transmitted pathogen; ceftriaxone 250mg IM single dose, plus doxycycline 100mg BD for 10–14 days.
2. If due to chlamydia or other non-gonococcal organism; doxycycline 100mg BD for 10–14 days or ofloxacin 200mg BD for 14 days.
3. For epididymo-orchitis probably due to enteric pathogens; ofloxacin 200mg BD for 14 days or ciprofloxacin 500mg BD for 10 days.

Sexual partners

Partner notification and treatment is recommended for all patients with infection secondary to gonorrhoea, chlamydia and for indeterminate aetiology.

Relevant literature

Clinical Effectiveness Group, British Association for Sexual Health and HIV (2010). *United Kingdom national guideline for the management of epididymo-orchitis*.

CASE 51 Diabetes

INFORMATION FOR THE DOCTOR

Name	Alan Tiffin
Age	63
Social and family history	• Married • Occupation: pub owner
Medical history	• Eczema • Essential hypertension • Vasectomy
Current medication	• Diprobase ointment BD • Perindopril 2mg OD
Blood tests FBC U&E LFTs Plasma glucose Total cholesterol Plasma HDL cholesterol Plasma cholesterol/ HDL ratio Free T$_4$ TSH PSA Recent BP BMI	*Blood tests done recently* HB 13.5 (13.5–18.0) WBC 9.4 × 10^9/L (4.0–11.0) Plt 296 × 10^9/L (150–400) Na 134mmol/L (135–146) K 3.8mmol/L (3.2–5.1) Ur 2.2mmol/L (1.7–8.3) Cr 62μmol/L (62–106) T. bilirubin 5μmol/L (0–21) ALT 21IU/L (0–41) Alk phos 118IU/L (40–129) 7.4 (fasting) 6.0mmol/L (2.8–5.0) 1.2mmol/L 5 14.8pmol/L 1.4 (0.3–4.2) 0.17ng/ml (0–4.0) 130/78 30

INFORMATION FOR THE PATIENT

You are Alan Tiffin, a 63-year-old man and father of two grown-up boys. You live with your wife and own a pub. You have been feeling tired for the past few weeks and were advised routine blood tests. Bloods last year were normal. You are here to discuss blood results.

Information to reveal if asked

General information about yourself:

- You are married and live with your wife. You own and run a pub. You work long hours, it is a family business and your wife and two sons help you to run it.

- You admit you lead an unhealthy lifestyle; being a pub owner, you can consume up to two bottles of wine a day, and occasionally vodka. Average alcohol consumption 100–140 units a week.

- You smoke 10 cigarettes/day. You do not have much time for active exercise. Your diet is usually the pub food. You love steak/red meat, fish and chips with not much green vegetables.

- You do not do much exercise.

Further details about your condition:

- You have a family history of heart disease. Both your older brothers have diabetes. Your father died of a heart attack at 65. One of your brothers has angina, had a stent put in a few months ago and is on statins. Your other brother has diabetes, is on tablets.

- You have been feeling very tired lately. There is no change in your bowel habit or appetite. You have been drinking a lot and having frequent urination. You are unable to comment on your weight, haven't noticed much.

Your ideas:

- You think this could be diabetes. You have spoken to your brother who has the condition and he had similar complaints before they did a blood test.

- You are realistic, you know you have an unhealthy lifestyle and are aware of the problems it may cause. You know about heart problems as your brother and father have had heart attack and stents. You will not be able to make many lifestyle changes.

Your concerns:

- You have heard stories about foot amputation and eye problems with diabetes and would rather commence on tablets to help you if you are a diabetic.

- You are not surprised to hear about your cholesterol and blood sugar results but worried if you could be at risk of having vision problems or foot problems.

Your expectations:

- You want to know the blood results and if you have diabetes.

Information to reveal if examined

- No examination required.

SUGGESTED APPROACH TO THE CONSULTATION

Targeted history taking:

- Take a detailed history of patient's lifestyle. This is to include his diet, activity levels or exercise. Also information regarding alcohol consumption and smoking status.

- Obtain details of tiredness symptoms. Any red flags to be excluded.

- Family history is important.

Clinical management:

- Highlight the fasting blood glucose of 7.4 which, together with his symptoms of tiredness, probably point to a diagnosis of diabetes. However, it is rare to make the diagnosis of diabetes based on a single test result, even when symptomatic, so it is best to arrange a second blood test (either HbA1c or fasting glucose) to confirm the diagnosis. Also take the opportunity to arrange a urine specimen for ACR.

- Explain the condition of type 2 diabetes, its management and prognosis.

- Check patient's understanding about the condition.

- Discuss BMI (currently 30) and insulin resistance. Encourage weight loss. Make the patient aware of structured educational programmes such as Diabetes2gether, to which he will be referred once his diagnosis is confirmed. Encourage regular exercise.

- Discuss his smoking and offer referral to a smoking cessation clinic.

- Highlight the importance of the above lifestyle changes in management of diabetes.

- Discuss his cholesterol results and how it could be improved through a low-calorie, Mediterranean-style diet and more exercise. If lifestyle measures fail to achieve targets of TC<4 or LDL<2, then a statin may be needed.

- Address his concerns about foot problems or eye complications.

- Offer treatment options and arrange suitable follow-ups.

Interpersonal skills:

This case tests the doctor's ability to confirm to a patient the bad news he already suspects, and to provide support, education and advice. The challenge in this case is the ability to prioritise what needs to be done first; a long journey begins with the first step. Discuss with the patient how he feels about the news; what he understands to be the problems; what support he needs from you (and the practice) and explain how the practice team will co-ordinate his care so we can help him to improve his health and his lifestyle. A good GP displays empathy, caring and encouragement.

Good communication with the patient:

- checks patient's understanding of the condition and addresses his concerns.

- avoids jargon and reassures patient that timely management and good control would minimise complications.

BACKGROUND KNOWLEDGE REQUIRED FOR THIS CASE

What issues should be covered at initial and review consultations for type 2 diabetes?

All of the following are unlikely to be covered in a single appointment and may need to be covered over several consultations:

- **Diabetes education**: offer structured education at diagnosis and at least annually thereafter, preferably through a structured diabetes education programme.
- **Diet and lifestyle**: dietary history should be obtained and advice should be provided by a person with expertise in nutrition (such as a registered dietician).
  - Encourage weight loss if the person is overweight.
  - Encourage smoking cessation if the person smokes.
  - Encourage regular exercise.
- **Glucose control**: review the person's HbA1c level and agree an appropriate target level:
  - If managed by diet alone or by one drug, a target HbA1c of 6.5% (48mmol/mol) is generally recommended. If the person requires more intensive treatment, a target of less than 7.5% (59mmol/mol) is generally recommended. If HbA1c is within target, recheck within 6 months.
- **Blood pressure (BP)**: measure BP at least once a year in a person without previously diagnosed hypertension or renal disease and every 4–6 months in a person who is taking antihypertensive treatment or has renal disease. If there is kidney, eye or cerebrovascular damage, the target BP is less than 130/80mmHg. For others, the target BP is less than 140/80mmHg. If the person is on antihypertensive therapy at diagnosis, only make changes if BP is poorly controlled or if current treatment is inappropriate because of microvascular complications or metabolic problems.
- **Assess the need for lipid-modification therapy**: most people with type 2 diabetes should be taking a statin. If taking a statin, aim for total cholesterol <4mmol/L or low-density lipoprotein cholesterol <2mmol/L. If lipids are within target, repeat assessment annually.

Assess for complications of diabetes:

- **Feet**: examine the feet at diagnosis and at least annually thereafter.

- **Eyes**: ensure that all people with diabetes are referred for retinal screening at diagnosis as part of a formal screening programme. All people should have annual retinal screening, or more frequent screening if significant eye disease is present.

- **Kidneys**: assess for the presence of kidney disease at diagnosis and at least annually thereafter.

- **Neuropathy**: assess for the presence of neuropathy (including erectile dysfunction in men) at diagnosis and annually thereafter.

For information on diagnosing and step-up treatment of diabetes, see www.gp-update.co.uk/assets/docs/gp%20update%20handbook%20autumn%20 2014%20winter%202015%20diabetes.pdf

Summary of NICE guidelines for diabetes (CG87, 2009)

1. Patient education and dietary advice are crucial. Initial body weight loss target is 5–10% for an overweight person.
2. Assessment of blood glucose control HbA1c is 6.5% but individual HbA1c may vary. Monitor 2–6-monthly until stable, then 6-monthly once blood glucose level is stable.
3. Self-monitoring should be available to those on insulin, on oral hypoglycaemics, to assess changes in blood glucose related to medications and lifestyle, to monitor during intercurrent illness and to ensure safety during activities including driving.
4. Medication.

Author's interpretation of NICE guidelines on type 2 diabetes

1. Start lifestyle interventions.
2. Metformin or sulphonylurea if not overweight or unable to take metformin.
3. Metformin + sulphonylurea **or**
   metformin + gliptin or glitazone if not able to take sulphonylurea.
4. Metformin + sulphonylurea + insulin **or**
   can add gliptin/glitazone **or**
   exenatide if insulin unacceptable.
   Intensify insulin regimen/add insulin.
5. *Management of blood lipids*

Review cardiovascular risk and features of metabolic syndrome/waist circumference.

High-risk patients include:

- Overweight patients
- Hypertensive >140/80mmHg or on medications (antihypertensives)
- Smokers

- High risk lipid profile
- History of cardiovascular disease
- Family history of cardiovascular disease

Treat to achieve total cholesterol <4.0mmol/L. Can increase simvastatin to 80mg daily; can intensify therapy with effective statin or ezetimibe.

Monitor 1–3 months after starting therapy, monitor annually.

6. *Anti-thrombotic therapy*

Advice from SIGN *Guidelines on the Management of Diabetes* (2010) is that aspirin should not be used for primary prevention in people with diabetes.

7. *Blood pressure management*

In target organ damage (kidney, eye or cerebrovascular) set target at <130/80mmHg; for others, aim for <140/80mmHg.

8. *Kidney damage*

Monitor annually regardless of nephropathy. Arrange ACR estimation, serum creatinine and GFR.

Abnormal ACR= >2.5mg/mmol for men and >3.5mg/mmol for women.

If diabetic nephropathy confirmed, offer ACE inhibitor/ARB and maintain BP <130/80mmHg.

9. *Eye screening*

Screen at or around time of diagnosis. Eye surveillance annually.

10. *Neuropathic pain management*

Assess every year. If symptoms uncontrolled offer tricyclic drugs; also can consider opiate analgesia. Neuropathic complications like gastroparesis, erectile dysfunction and foot problems to be kept in mind.

11. Look out for depression.

CASE 52 Gout

INFORMATION FOR THE DOCTOR

This is a telephone consultation.

Name	Samuel Yates
Age	62
Social and family history	• He lives with his wife. They have no children • Non-smoker • Alcohol: beer 3–4 cans a day, can be more on weekends
Past medical history	• Hypertension • Gout • Osteoarthritis
Current medication	• Ramipril 10mg OD • Omeprazole 20mg OD • Diclofenac 50mg TDS/PRN
Blood tests Total cholesterol Triglycerides LDL Fasting glucose level FBC U&E BP BMI	*Blood tests done last week* 7.3mmol/L (2.8–5) 1.8mmol/L 5.4mmol/L (0–3) 5.0mmol/L WNL (with normal limits) Sodium 140mmol/L (135–145) Potassium 4.2mmol/L (3.2–5.0) Creatinine 87µmol/L (44–80) Serum urate 0.62mmol/L (0.2–0.42) 152/97mmHg 38

INFORMATION FOR THE PATIENT

You are 62-year-old Samuel Yates. You live with your wife in a two-bedroom flat. You were a postman, retired two years ago. You now have a relaxed lifestyle. You spend most of your time at home watching television, occasionally do some housework and DIY.

Your evenings are spent at a local pub where you catch up with old friends.

Your gout has flared up again. Having seen a locum at the practice last week who requested blood tests, you are making this phone call to your usual doctor to get your blood test results and to request a prescription for some painkillers.

Information to reveal if asked
General information about yourself:
- You are now retired, live with your wife and enjoy life with your friends. You have few hobbies, spend your days doing chores around the house and watching TV.

Further details about your condition:
- You have had another flare-up of gout and need a prescription of diclofenac. You have been otherwise well and were last seen in surgery 18 months ago for a sore throat.
- You have had gout for the last 5 years but progressively getting worse with more frequent attacks. You have had four attacks this year. Diclofenac works well. You usually have it with food and are able to tolerate it well.
- It is usually your right big toe which gets inflamed and painful but this time it is both big toes and right ankle which have been affected. You once used a drug called colchicine but diclofenac works better.
- You are unable to do much exercise due to your knee osteoarthritis and recurrent attacks of gout. You were doing a lot of walking when you delivered letters but all that is a thing of the past.
- You enjoy your beer and admit that your alcohol intake is high, especially at the weekends.

Your ideas:
- You believe that gout is a familial condition as your father had it too.
- You were advised regarding diet and alcohol and have made significant changes to your food habits. You have cut out red meat completely and now eat fish and chicken. You loved steak and sausages but now hardly consume them. You love your beer and will try to cut down.

Your concerns:

- You are worried about your mobility if these attacks continue to get worse in frequency and severity. Your father was nearly immobile due to severe gout and weight problems. He died of a heart attack. He was 58 years old when he died. He was overweight. You do not know more details about his health problems.

Your expectations:

- A drug called allopurinol was offered 6 months ago which will prevent these attacks and now you would like to consider it.
- You want a prescription for diclofenac and also this drug which will prevent further attacks.

Other information

You had not had a blood test in the last 2 years; the locum you saw last week said this would be needed before the new drug could be considered.

BP 152/97mmHg

BMI 38

SUGGESTED APPROACH TO THE CONSULTATION

Targeted history taking:

- Obtain details about his gout, flare-up, severity of symptoms and impact on life.
- What is his understanding about gout and the flare-ups?
- Ask about diet (consumption of purine-rich food), number of alcohol units per week, and exercise taken (type, duration, intensity, frequency).
- Explore whether the patient understands the link between diet, alcohol, gout, BP and CV risk.
- What has he been told about allopurinol? Is he aware of the drug, side-effects and time it needs to be commenced?

Targeted examination:

- Examination is not needed in this case but interpretation of blood results and BMI finding need to be addressed.

Clinical management:

- Address patient's concerns about the frequency and severity of attacks of gout. Discuss importance of diet, exercise and weight reduction which would play an important part in management of his condition.
- Discuss role of allopurinol and time to start the drug. Inform him that the acute attack needs to subside before allopurinol could be considered.
- Offer naproxen as an alternative to diclofenac. COX-2 inhibitors and other NSAIDs have a higher risk of MI compared to naproxen.
- Discuss blood results, high cholesterol and high BMI, their relation to gout and cardiovascular risks.
- Arrange suitable follow-up to review gout and cardiovascular assessment.

BACKGROUND KNOWLEDGE REQUIRED FOR THIS CASE

Gout

Gout is associated with serious comorbidity and increased risk of cardiovascular disease.

A clinical diagnosis can be made when typical features of inflammation affect the first metatarsophalyngeal joint. First-line medical treatment options for acute gout are an NSAID or low-dose colchicine.

Long-term management requires full patient education, dealing with any modifiable risk factors (such as overweight or obesity, chronic diuretic use).

Prevalence of gout is rising because of an ageing population, increasing prevalence of metabolic syndrome and possibly dietary changes.

Clinically important risk factors for gout:

- Male sex
- Older age
- Genetic factors (mainly reduced excretion of urate)
- Obesity (reduced excretion of urate)
- Hypertension (reduced excretion of urate)
- Hyperlipidaemia (reduced excretion of urate)
- Loop and thiazide diuretics (reduced excretion of urate)
- Chronic kidney disease (reduced excretion of urate)
- Osteoarthritis (enhanced crystal formation)
- Dietary factors (increased production of uric acid):
  - Excess purine-rich foods, fructose, sugar-sweetened soft drinks
  - Excess alcohol consumption, particularly beer

Gout is increasingly being viewed as more than just a joint disease. Comorbidity including hypertension, hyperlipidaemia, CKD, diabetes, congestive heart failure and ischaemic heart disease is common and often unrecognised and undertreated.

Treatment

Acute

British Society for Rheumatology and American College of Rheumatology guidelines suggest using a fast-acting NSAID, such as naproxen.

There was also a 38% reduction in those treated with low-dose colchicine (1.2mg initially, followed by 0.6mg).

Corticosteroids provide a further treatment option.

Urate-lowering drugs

The most commonly used drug is allopurinol. It should be started at low dose (usual increments monthly until serum uric acid is below 360μmol/L). The maximum permitted dose of allopurinol in UK is 900mg per day. An alternative is febuxostat. Treatment is lifelong.

Relevant literature

Roddy, E, Mallen, CD and Doherty, M (2013) **Gout** (Clinical Review). *BMJ*, **347**: F5648.